54.50

The Clinical roots of the
schizophrenia concept : translations of
seminal European contributions on

The clinical roots of the schizophrenia concept

The clinical roots of the schizophrenia concept

TRANSLATIONS OF SEMINAL EUROPEAN
CONTRIBUTIONS ON SCHIZOPHRENIA

Edited by

JOHN CUTTING
Consultant Psychiatrist, Bethlem and Maudsley Hospitals, London

M. SHEPHERD
Professor of Epidemiological Psychiatry
Institute of Psychiatry, London

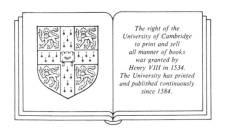

The right of the
University of Cambridge
to print and sell
all manner of books
was granted by
Henry VIII in 1534.
The University has printed
and published continuously
since 1584.

CAMBRIDGE UNIVERSITY PRESS

Cambridge

London New York New Rochelle

Melbourne Sydney

Published by the Press Syndicate of the University of Cambridge
The Pitt Building, Trumpington Street, Cambridge CB2 1RP
32 East 57th Street, New York, NY 10022, USA
10 Stamford Road, Oakleigh, Melbourne 3166, Australia

First published 1987

Printed in Great Britain at the University Press, Cambridge

British Library cataloguing in publication data

The clinical roots of the schizophrenia concept: translations of
    seminal European contributions on schizophrenia.

    1. Schizophrenia
    I. Cutting, J.   II. Shepherd, Michael, 1923–
    616.89'82   RC514

Library of Congress cataloging in publication data

The Clinical roots of the schizophrenia concept.

    Includes index.
    1. Schizophrenia – Collected works.   I. Cutting, John
    II. Shepherd, Michael, 1923– .   [DNLM: 1. Schizophrenia – collected
    works.   WM 203 C6413]
    RC514.C57 1986   616.89'82   86-11766

ISBN 0521 26635 1

PN

Contents

	Preface	vii
	Introduction	1
Part I	**German-language contributions**	11
A	*The clinical and psychological analysis of dementia praecox*	
	Emil Kraepelin Dementia praecox	13
	Otto Diem The simple dementing form of dementia praecox	25
	Otto Gross Dementia sejunctiva	35
	Erwin Stransky Towards an understanding of certain symptoms of dementia praecox	37
	Wilhelm Weygandt Critical comments on the psychology of dementia praecox	42
	Joseph Berze Primary insufficiency of mental activity	51
B	*The introduction of the term schizophrenia*	
	Eugen Bleuler The prognosis of dementia praecox: the group of schizophrenias	59
C	*The evolution of the concept of schizophrenia*	
	Karl Kleist Alogical thought disorder: an organic manifestation of the schizophrenic psychological deficit	75
	Gustav Störring Perplexity	79
	Ludwig Binswanger Extravagance, perverseness, manneristic behaviour and schizophrenia	83
	Paul Matussek Studies in delusional perception	89
	Gerhardt Schmidt A review of the German literature on delusion between 1914 and 1939	104
D	*The current state of psychopathology*	
	Werner Janzarik The crisis in psychopathology	135
Part II	**French-language contributions**	145
	Philippe Chaslin Discordant insanity	147

Ernest Dupré and **Jean Logre** Confabulatory delusional states   159
Paul Sérieux and **Joseph Capgras** Misinterpretative delusional
states   169
Gaétan Gatian de Clérambault Psychoses of passion   182
Eugene Minkowski The essential disorder underlying
schizophrenia and schizophrenic thought   188
Jacques Lacan The case of Aimée, or self-punitive
paranoia   213
Index   227

Preface

The purpose of this collection of translations is to acquaint contemporary students of schizophrenia with some of the seminal works on the subject. While the literature on the subject of schizophrenia continues to grow at an enormous rate, the quality of some recent work suffers in some measure because the pressure to publish discourages workers from placing their own findings in historical context. The editors hope that by consulting papers in this collection, contemporary students will be able to enrich and broaden their own contributions.

This book would not have been possible without expert translators, and we should like to thank both Miss Helen Marshall, ex-librarian of the Institute of Psychiatry, and Dr Ralph Emery, formerly consultant psychiatrist at Brookwood Hospital, Surrey, for their labours.

Some of the papers are not translated in full. This is indicated in the text by the usual convention – . . .

J. Cutting
M. Shepherd

Introduction

The concept of dementia praecox or schizophrenia has undergone marked changes since its original formulations by Kraepelin and Bleuler at the turn of the century. At that time it was regarded as a brain disease differing from other neurological conditions only in the tantalising absence of any definite observable pathology at post-mortem.

Between the two World Wars a marked divergence of opinion developed concerning its nature. Different countries, different schools of thought and various eminent psychiatrists all had their own viewpoints, most of them at variance with Kraepelin's original concept. There was a shift away from an organic towards a social formulation, attributable in some measure to the absence of detectable brain pathology and the undoubted social deterioration which was out of keeping with any intellectual decline.

In the 1950s and 1960s despite the appearance of new psychotropic drugs, the psychological and social formulations were so influential that some authorities even suggested that schizophrenia was an artefact, a construct designed to label misfits as mad, and that the early clinicians had been duped into thinking that their patients were ill. By the 1970s it became clear that this was too extreme a view, and various workers and international bodies began to develop reliable but empirical ways of defining the condition. Nonetheless, there was still no identifiable cerebral disorder to validate these definitions.

In the last few years, however, it has become apparent that the absence of gross brain pathology does not in itself eliminate an organic basis for schizophrenia. More subtle disorders, exemplified by neurotransmitter abnormalities or a physiological imbalance between the activity of the two hemispheres have come to the fore and are attracting the attention of many neuroscientists working in the field.

In retrospect, it is now apparent that Kraepelin, his contemporaries and immediate successors, who were so often vilified by the 'anti-psychiatrists' and their sympathisers, deserve to be re-read in the light of the advances in biological psychiatry and the growth in neuropsychological knowledge of the last decade. The purpose of this collection is to acquaint contemporary students of schizophrenia with the views of their European predecessors in the earlier part of the century, not merely as a historical exercise in praise of famous men, but to show how the descriptions and psychological speculations of these clinicians have anticipated contemporary formulations. Each of the extracts translated here has been chosen either for its contemporary importance or for its relevance to current notions of schizophrenia.

The first section contains translations of work by Kraepelin, Diem, Gross, Stransky, Weygandt and Berze. Kraepelin's article is the first account in the literature of dementia praecox, the condition which Bleuler renamed the schizophrenias. Kraepelin's description of dementia praecox in the 1913 edition of his textbook was translated into English in 1919, but this very first account, succinct in form and bold in conception, deserves to be more widely known.

Simple schizophrenia, as described in Diem's article, has been something of a diagnostic enigma ever since Bleuler included it alongside the more obvious varieties. It is rarely diagnosed these days in Europe or America and many psychiatrists have recommended that the concept be abandoned (Stone *et al.*, 1968). However, there are several pointers in the recent literature to its diagnostic usefulness, and a case can be made for its resurrection. For example, schizophrenia is often regarded as a spectrum of disorders which include certain types of abnormal personality as well as a core group with frank psychosis (Rosenthal *et al.*, 1968). The link between psychotic individuals and certain non-psychotic eccentrics has been established by showing that both may emanate from the same genetic stock (Parnas *et al.*, 1982). What these two types of individual share, according to Siever & Gunderson (1983), is 'social isolation and suspiciousness' and, in particular, an autistic way of life. The simple schizophrenia of Diem and Bleuler can thus be seen as an early attempt to identify a schizophrenic psychological profile in non-psychotic but schizoid individuals. Another recent trend in the direction of Diem's concept is the recognition of similarities between *infantile autism*, particularly in its milder form, *Asperger's syndrome*, a personality type which resembles autism in certain ways, *schizophrenia* itself, and *schizoid personality*. Autism has hitherto been regarded by most authorities (e.g. Rutter, 1985) as quite distinct from schizophrenia, but this is now being questioned by investigators who have noted that the latter condition can supervene on the former (Howells & Guirguis, 1984). Further, the psychological profiles of autism (Rutter, 1985), Asperger's syndrome (Wing, 1981) schizophrenia (Cutting, 1985) and schizoid personality (Wolff & Chick, 1980) show many similarities. Simple schizophrenia can thus be regarded as an early description of a developmental disorder of thinking and feeling which does not progress to a frank psychosis. Diem recognised that such individuals frequently came to the notice of the forensic services, a point also noted in the case of Asperger's syndrome by Mawson *et al.* (1985), and in the case of schizoid individuals by Chick *et al.* (1986).

Consciousness and its pathological varieties constituted a common topic of scientific interest in the first two decades of the century, but from the 1920s, however, the advent of behaviourism as a mainstream model of psychology in the Anglo-American world discouraged any discussion of the role of altered consciousness in schizophrenia until recently. In the last decade, however, several authors have reintroduced the concept to explain some of the symptoms of the condition. Two articles translated here, those by Gross and Berze, directly examine the possibility that disturbed consciousness might underlie many of the phenomena seen in schizophrenia. According to Gross, there is a general breakdown in the cerebral processes responsible for generating consciousness. Berze indicated how this might explain such symptoms as depersonalisation, split personality and personality deterioration. In the past 10 years several workers have come to stress the importance of disturbed consciousness in schizophrenia. Frith (1979), for example, has proposed that: 'the symptoms of schizophrenia can be interpreted as a result of a defect in the mechanism that controls and limits the contents of consciousness. This defect can be understood as excessive self-awareness'. Jaynes (1976), on the other hand, has suggested that schizophrenics might have an unusually restricted consciousness. Nasrallah (1982) has speculated on whether some of the characteristic features of schizophrenia, notably the belief that thoughts and feelings are alien and controlled from outside, might arise as a result of excessive awareness by one hemisphere of the activity of the other. Because of the relationship between them, he argued, the dominant left hemisphere would not appreciate that the source of this increased activity was in the right hemisphere and would attribute it instead to an external agent.

The article by Stransky shows remarkable insight into the most characteristic of all schizophrenic features, the dissociation between and within mental functions. This is also stressed by Bleuler and in the paper by Minkowski. There is a topical flavour to Stransky's speculation on an imbalance, an 'intrapsychic ataxia' as he calls it, between the noo-psyche (intellectual side of life) and the thymo-psyche (emotional side of life). It was not until the 1950s, however, that the role of the right hemisphere in nonverbal perception and communication was appreciated and the late 1960s before the effects of hemisphere disconnection were recognised. In the last 10 or 15 years a large literature has sprung up concerning the possible relevance of hemisphere imbalance to schizophrenia (Gur, 1978; Flor-Henry, 1983; Cutting, 1985), and Stransky's speculations now appear remarkably prescient in the light of recent neuropsychological research on the lateralisation of cerebral functions.

Weygandt's article touches on a number of principles concerning the nature of schizophrenia, which were generally ignored for most of the century, but are now more or less established truths. He states, first, that schizophrenia is a disease of the brain, a statement which most North American psychiatrists have disputed until recently (Henn & Nasrallah, 1982). As a corollory, Weygandt is particularly critical of the attempts of Freud and subsequent psychoanalysts to regard schizophrenia as a neurosis, akin to hysteria, related causally to such factors as early life experiences, particularly the exposure to ambiguous and inconsistent child rearing, the effects of life events and various types of family environment. Little support has been provided for any of these hypotheses and Weygandt's position with regard to schizophrenia has been supported by most recent studies (e.g. MacMillan *et al.*, 1986).

The second section contains only one paper, that by Bleuler in which he first used the term schizophrenia. This too, has never been translated into English although his monograph, published three years later, was translated in 1950. The present article is, however, a useful synopsis of his larger work, and indicates the development as well as the origin of ideas on schizophrenia.

The third section contains articles by Kleist, Störring, Binswanger, Matussek and Schmidt. These were all written between 1930 and 1960, and show the divergence of opinion which developed concerning the nature of schizophrenia, even within German-speaking countries. Schmidt's comprehensive review on delusions illustrates well the richness and variety of psychiatric thought which was current in Germany between the two World Wars.

Kleist represents one extreme of this spectrum of ideas, but one which is undergoing a revival in recent years, particularly among North American neurologists such as Geschwind (Geschwind & Galaburda, 1985) and Cummings (1985), who all regard organic psychiatry as a branch of neurology. Kleist's concern with the similarities between the language and thought of schizophrenics and those of subjects with definite temporal or frontal lobe damage has also a modern counterpart among psychiatrists like Flor-Henry (1983) who regard the psychoses associated with temporal lobe epilepsy as a possible model of schizophrenia. Finally, Kleist's interest in the structure of language and thought in schizophrenia has been revived during the past decade, when several linguists (Chaika, 1974; LeCours & Vanier-Clément, 1976; Brown, 1977) have conducted careful analysis of the material and have compared the abnormalities with those found in aphasia from a known focal lesion.

If Kleist is located at the organic end of the spectrum of views on schizophrenia, Binswanger is at the other extreme. His existential analysis of the personal meaning of certain schizophrenic symptoms may appear far-fetched and fanciful to modern readers, but it may be recalled that only 25 years ago Laing's (1959) *The Divided Self* captured the imagination of countless non-medical professionals involved in caring for schizophrenics. Laing borrowed freely from Binswanger, and, by incorporating social and psychoanalytical components, made Binswanger's idea more appealing and less turgid. A strictly existential account of schizophrenia has little support nowadays, but elements of Binswanger's approach are still to be found outside the main psychiatric and psychological journals and in imaginative literature.

Perplexity, the topic of Störring's article, is rarely discussed in the Anglo-American literature, except as a diagnostic feature of non-schizophrenic functional psychoses such as cycloid psychosis (Perris, 1974). There is no psychological literature on the symptom, nor are its links with schizophrenia as clear as Störring appears to believe. Nevertheless, it is a common and relatively uninvestigated phenomenon and merits more attention.

Matussek and his teacher Conrad (1958) were among the first to recognise the importance of a disorder of perception in schizophrenia. Neither Kraepelin nor Bleuler regarded a perceptual disorder as part of the psychological deficit, and delusional perception, despite being recognised as a central feature of schizophrenia, had been regarded as a disorder of thinking rather than of perception (see Gruhle's account in Schmidt's article, page 106). Matussek appreciated that Gestalt psychology provided a broader model of perception than that permitted by the associationist or behavioural schools, and one which might explain at least the early stages of schizophrenia. Since that time several psychologists have followed this lead and there are now a number of robust experiments showing that schizophrenics are especially impaired in their *Gestalt* appreciation in a perceptual task (Schwartz Place & Gilmore, 1980; Frith *et al.*, 1983).

The fourth section also contains a single article, that by Janzarik, one of the most eminent contemporary German psychiatrists. Its content differs from the others, and it is included as a concise statement of the present state of Central European research in the field of psychopathology. The paper is based on a lecture given when the anti-psychiatry movement in Germany was at its height. It can be read both as an apologia for much of the material of this book and as a plea for the continuation of psychopathological research.

The final section contains articles by French psychiatrists – Chaslin, Dupré & Logre, Sérieux & Capgras, de Clérambault, Minkowski and Lacan. The views of Kraepelin and Bleuler have never been wholly accepted in France, where a somewhat idiosyncratic system of classification exists (Pichot, 1982). The French concept of functional psychosis consists in a narrowly defined category of schizophrenia, similar to the concept of the hebephrenic subgroup only, and a number of discrete psychoses, which replace the more customary concept of paranoid schizophrenia.

Chaslin's *'discordant insanity'*, a term which never became popular, even in France, is very similar to the notion of hebephrenic schizophrenia. All his four subgroups of 'discordant insanity' exhibit marked thought disorder and affective flattening, the two prominent features of the hebephrenic type. In recent years there has been a tendency to pay more attention to subgroups of schizophrenia, e.g. to divide the condition into familial and sporadic forms (Winokur *et al.*, 1974). Further, the familial variety tends to present with hebephrenic features and the sporadic to have a variety of environmental causes and paranoid features (Kendler & Hays, 1982). Such findings may give some support to the French tradition of restricting the concept of schizophrenia to the hebephrenic variety, represented here by Chaslin's 'discordant insanity'.

Dupré & Logre's account of *'délires d'imagination'*, translated here as *'confabulatory delusional states'*, illustrates another characteristic trend in French psychiatry, i.e. to subdivide paranoid states according to the mental function which appears most affected. Hitherto Anglo-American workers have tended to eschew the use of discrete diagnostic labels for a functional psychosis other than schizophrenia, mania, depressive psychosis and possibly schizoaffective psychosis and to pay relatively little attention to the origin and development of delusions per se. These habits are changing. There is a small but growing interest in what Winokur (1977) has called delusional disorder, pure delusional states without any other characteristics of schizophrenia or affective disorder. There are also several research projects in progress (e.g. Garety, 1985) examining the nature of belief in deluded subjects. A 'selective disorder of the faculty of creative imagination', as suggested by Dupré & Logre, may well prove to be one route for the development or maintenance of a delusion.

Sérieux & Capgras' *'délire d'interpretation'*, translated here as a *misinterpretative delusional state*, is an even more persuasive account of how delusions can arise, in this case solely through false reasoning. There are numerous studies examining the role and nature of disordered reasoning in schizophrenia. Two recent investigations (Robertson & Taylor, 1985; Liddle, 1986) found that although deteriorated and hebephrenic schizophrenics had marked deficits in concept attainment tasks, otherwise well-preserved deluded subjects performed no worse than normal controls. This might suggest that false reasoning is not a common cause of delusional development, but may play a part in a subgroup of deluded subjects, as suggested by Sérieux & Capgras.

De Clérambault's name as the originator of the term erotomania is well known, though his writings on the matter have not, to our knowledge, been translated before. The general concept of *'psychoses passionelles'*, translated here as *psychoses of passion*, is recognised in the psychoanalytical literature and under other names has been discussed in the general psychological literature. Behaviourists, for example, have attributed delusional formation to excessive anxiety or drive (Mednick, 1958; Broen & Storms, 1966). The recent attempts to modify delusions by means of cognitive therapy (e.g. Hartman & Cashman, 1983) has highlighted the importance of emotion in the maintenance of a delusion, though not necessarily in its causation.

Minkowski brought a wholly individual approach to schizophrenia, and it is difficult to place him neatly within a particular school of thought, or even to say at which end of the organic-psychosocial spectrum he should be placed. One of the editors of this book, however, considers that his ideas can only now be seen as providing insight into the nature of schizophrenia (Cutting, 1985). Although sometimes expressed in rather poetic fashion and drawing heavily on

Bergson's philosophy, his concepts are original. Five points stand out. First, there is the notion of autism, which he places above most other phenomena, and to which he gives even more emphasis than Bleuler. Secondly there is his careful analysis of the difference between intellectual dementia, as observed in true organic conditions, and schizophrenic dementia; he concludes that it is common sense or pragmatic knowledge of the world which suffers most in schizophrenia. Thirdly, there is his notion of the schizophrenics' pre-occupation with space and their relative neglect of the temporal aspects of their life. Fourthly, there is his astute observation that the schizophrenic is over-intellectual and over-abstract in his thinking to the detriment of any psychological, emotional and social considerations. The only modern counterpart to these ideas is the current trend, as mentioned above, to link autism, Asperger's syndrome, schizoid personality and schizophrenia. Finally, his list of what he and his wife termed 'atrophied' and 'hypertrophied' aspects of thought almost exactly mirrors the lists of those functions or aspects of the world which are selectively dealt with by each hemisphere (Bogen, 1969). In this way Minkowski, like Stransky, foreshadows the present interest in cerebral hemispheric imbalance (Cutting, 1985).

Lacan's article is included as a particularly insightful and well formulated example of a psychogenic psychosis. The concept of a psychogenic or reactive psychosis, one entirely attributable to personality disorder or adverse life events without any genetic or organic abnormalities, has been a recurrent theme throughout the history of psychiatry. Whether Lacan is correct in the precise formulation of the psychological mechanism in his case is open to doubt, but the concept will continue to survive until such time as the organic and genetic causes of psychosis are clearly established.

As a group, therefore, these 19 papers merit careful study not only for their historical interest but for their contemporary relevance to the study and understanding of schizophrenia.

References

Bogen, J. E. (1969) The other side of the brain. *Bulletin of the Los Angeles Neurological Society* **34**, 135–62.

Broen, W. E. & Storms, L. H. (1966) Lawful disorganisation: the process underlying the schizophrenic syndrome. *Psychological Review* **73**, 265–79.

Brown, J. (1977) *Mind, Brain and Consciousness: the Neuropsychology of Cognition.* New York: Academic Press.

Chaika, E. (1974) A linguist looks at "schizophrenic language". *Brain and Language* **1**, 257–76.

Chick, J. *et. al.* (1986) Schizoid personality and antisocial behaviour. *Psychological Medicine* (In Press).

Conrad, K. (1958) *Die Beginnende Schizophrenie*. Stuttgart: G. Thieme.

Cummings, J. (1985) *Neuropsychiatry*. New York: Academic Press.

Cutting, J. (1985) *The Psychology of Schizophrenia*. Edinburgh: Churchill Livingstone.

Flor-Henry, P. (1983) *Cerebral Basis of Psychopathology*. Bristol: John Wright.

Frith, C. D. (1979) Consciousness, information processing and schizophrenia. *British Journal of Psychiatry* **134**, 225–35.

Frith, C. D., Stevens, M., Johnstone, E. C., Owens, D. C. & Crow T. J. (1983) Integration of schematic faces and other complex objects in schizophrenia. *Journal of Nervous and Mental Diseases* **171**, 34–9.

Garety, P. (1985) Delusions: problems in definition and measurement. *British Journal of Medical Psychology* **58**, 25–34.

Geschwind N. & Galaburda, A. M. (1985) Cerebral lateralisation. *Archives of Neurology* **42**, 634–54.

Gur, R. E. (1978) Left hemisphere dysfunction and left hemisphere overactivation in schizophrenia. *Journal of Abnormal Psychology* **87**, 226–38.

Hartman, L. M. & Cashman, F. E. (1983) Cognitive-behavioural and psychopharmocological treatment of delusional symptoms: a preliminary report. *Behavioural Psychotherapy* **11**, 50–61.

Henn, F. A. & Nasrallah, H. A. (1982) (eds) *Schizophrenia as a Brain Disease*. New York: Oxford University Press.

Howells, J. G. & Guirguis, W. R. (1985) Childhood schizophrenia 20 years later. *Archives of General Psychiatry* **41**, 123–8.

Jaynes, J. (1976) *The Origin of Consciousness in the Breakdown of the Bicameral Mind*. Boston: Houghton Mifflin.

Kendler, K. S. & Hays, P. (1982) Familial and sporadic schizophrenia: a symptomatic, prognostic and E.E.G. comparison. *American Journal of Psychiatry* **139**, 1557–62.

Laing, R. D. (1959) *The Divided Self*. London: Tavistock.

LeCours, A. R. & Vanier-Clément, M. (1976) Schizophrenia and jargonaphasia. *Brain and Language* **3**, 516–65.

Liddle, P. F. (1986) Schizophrenic syndromes, cognitive performance and neurological dysfunction. *Psychological Medicine* (In Press).

MacMillan, J. F., Gold, A., Crow, T. J., Johnson, A.L. & Johnstone, E. C. (1986) Expressed emotion and relapse. *British Journal of Psychiatry* **148**, 133–43.

Mawson, D., Grounds, A. & Tantum, D. (1985) Violence and Asperger's syndrome: a case study. *British Journal of Psychiatry* **147**, 566–9.

Mednick, S. A. (1958) A learning theory approach to research in schizophrenia. *Psychological Bulletin* **55**, 316–27.

Nasrallah, H. A. (1982) Laterality and hemispheric dysfunction in schizophrenia. In *Schizophrenia as a Brain Disease* (ed. F. A. Henn & H. A. Nasrallah). New York: Oxford University Press.

Parnas, J., Schulsinger, F., Schulsinger, H., Mednick, S. A. & Teasdale, T. T. (1982). Behavioural precursors of schizophrenia spectrum. *Archives of General Psychiatry* **39**, 658–64.

Perris, C. (1974) A study of cycloid psychosis. *Acta Psychiatrica Scandinavica Supplement* 253.

Pichot, P. (1982) The diagnosis and classification of mental disorders in French-speaking countries. *Psychological Medicine* **12**, 475–92.

Robertson, G. & Taylor, P. J. (1985) Some cognitive correlates of schizophrenic illnesses. *Psychological Medicine* **15**, 81–98.

Rosenthal, D., Wender, P. H., Kety, S. S., Schulsinger, F., Welner, J. & Ostergaard, L. (1968). Schizophrenics' offspring reared in adoptive homes. In *The Transmission of Schizophrenia* (ed. D. Rosenthal & S. S. Kety). Oxford: Pergamon.

Rutter, M. (1985) Infantile autism and other pervasive developmental disorders. In *Child and Adolescent Psychiatry*, ed. M. Rutter & L. Hersov, 2nd edn. Oxford: Blackwell.

Schwartz Place, E. J. & Gilmore, G. C. (1980) Perceptual organization in schizophrenia. *Journal of Abnormal Psychology* **89**, 409–18.

Siever, L. J. & Gunderson, J. G. (1983) The search for a schizotypal personality: historical origins and current status. *Comprehensive Psychiatry* **24**, 199–212.

Stone, A. A., Hopkins, R., Mahnke, M. W., Shapiro, D. W. & Silverglate, H. A. (1968) Simple schizophrenia: syndrome or shibboleth. *American Journal of Psychiatry* **125**, 305–12.

Wing, L. (1981) Asperger's syndrome. *Psychological Medicine* **11**, 115–30.

Winokur, G. (1977) Delusional disorder (paranoia). *Comprehensive Psychiatry* **18**, 511–21.

Winokur, G., Morrison, J., Clancy, J. & Crowe, R. (1974) Iowa 500: the clinical and genetic distinction of hebephrenic and paranoid schizophrenia. *Journal of Nervous and Mental Diseases* **159**, 12–19.

Wolff, S. & Chick, J. (1980) Schizoid personality in childhood: a controlled follow-up study. *Psychological Medicine* **10**, 85–100.

I

German-language contributions

Emil Kraepelin (1856–1926)

Emil Kraepelin was born in a small village near the Baltic Sea, studied medicine in Würzburg and then, after short periods as a research assistant to the psychologist Wundt and to the neuropathologist and neuroanatomist Flechsig, he was appointed professor of Clinical Psychiatry in Munich, where he remained until his retirement.

He is widely regarded as a father of modern psychiatry, and is best known for his identification and careful description of dementia praecox. Although its name was later changed to schizophrenia, and although some subsequent psychiatrists have criticised Kraepelin for being too neurological in orientation, such criticisms are unfair and fail to appreciate the resilience of the concept which he developed. He was an organic psychiatrist by today's standards, but was far more sophisticated in his treatment of disease categories than many of his contemporaries who multiplied these categories too readily. He was also an acute observer of mental phenomena, and his notions about the essential psychological nature of dementia praecox have been overlooked by subsequent writers. The following extract is his first description of dementia praecox in the fifth edition of his textbook published in 1896. It has never been translated before.

Dementia praecox
E. Kraepelin (1896)
(Pages 426–41 of the 5th edition of *Psychiatrie*. Barth: Leipzig)

Dementia praecox is the name I have given to the development of a simple, fairly high-grade state of mental impairment accompanied by an acute or subacute mental disturbance.

The course of the illness may vary. We shall first consider those cases which are characterised by a restricted presentation of all the possible symptoms; many never come to the attention of the psychiatrist, nor are they attributed to morbid processes. The whole disturbance can be very gradual and the symptoms so ill-defined that relatives see them only as the result of an unfortunate development or perhaps a weakness in character. As a rule it gradually becomes apparent that the mental faculties of the patient are declining. He may still show the same or even greater industriousness, apply himself tirelessly to his books, engage in massive, inappropriate and indigestible reading or, occasionally, occupy himself with remote and difficult problems. In fact, however, he is no longer able to grasp anything correctly, to follow complicated arguments, or to concentrate his attention. He is distracted, his thoughts wander aimlessly, he dreams and broods without any real interest or recognisable aim and reads the same passage over and over again from start to finish without understanding it. He will make mistakes even in simple copying, by introducing variations, leaving some things out, and making arbitrary and inappropriate insertions. In the early stages we may find hypochondriacal complaints, self-reproach, fears for the future, and even transient ideas of persecution or of grandeur. Such disturbances, however, are usually vague and indefinite and do not develop further. Rarely, there may be hallucinations of sensations or voices. One such patient kept hearing sentences like the following:

> For we ourselves can always hope that we should let ourselves pay for other thoughts. For we want it ourselves, want to know it, who with us should let the swine torture to death. No, we ourselves are no longer so stupid and do not always bother if we should spare ourselves from drinking. For we play the fool and should let ourselves be tricked silly.

While saying this he seemed quite rational, laughed at such nonsense, thought he was ill and even went on working. From other accounts, however, he had clearly become less mentally competent, though hitherto he had been of higher than average intellectual ability.

In the early stages of this morbid disturbance memory remains basically intact. The patient retains throughout a store of knowledge, which in some cases is very extensive, and an excellent command of language. Some patients may still achieve a certain standard of rote learning, while others may take days to master a few words or proverbs. They are always, however, completely incapable of comprehending and developing new ideas. Individual components of experience are no longer connected; there is no interaction between them; they lead to no concepts, judgements or conclusions. In spite of the good memory retention, therefore, there is still an inevitable and progressive mental deterioration, the most striking features of which are the patient's inexplicable lack of judgement and the incoherence of all his thinking.

Consciousness remains unclouded; the patient is never disoriented in space or in his relationships, and not infrequently he is aware, with varying degrees of clarity, that his mental faculties are declining. He makes no further progress in his profession, passes no examinations, carries out no complicated mental tasks, and sets about things the wrong way round and in an aimless fashion. His intellectual horizon narrows; easy relationships with the outside world shrivel away. As a rule he gradually loses all interest in mental activities or mental stimulation, his thoughts move only in well-worn stereotyped grooves, and in the end he may be limited to mechanical activity – sawing wood, copying, gardening – often in sharp contrast to earlier ambitions, plans and hopes.

In the early stages mood is usually labile. We frequently encounter dejection, ill-humour or excitable disputatious behaviour; or there may be a sudden and groundless change from boisterousness with heightened self-esteem to an anxious sense of failure. At a later stage these mood swings are replaced by a degree of dullness which is only occasionally relieved by sudden, isolated outbursts. It is surprising how well the patient accepts his disabilities and failures. Although he admits that he has done many things in a topsy-turvy fashion, and has been 'very foolish', he is still quite pleased with his situation and is not worried about the future. He does not reflect upon his condition but lives from day to day, sometimes apathetically, at other times with a vague and sanguine expectation of some future good fortune.

In their actions patients show either great idleness and slackness or bear a childish, foolish stamp. Their will is unstable, with no independent force; at one moment they are stupidly obstinate, at the next suddenly docile and manageable. They neglect their personal appearance, live erratically, misplace objects of importance, forget their obligations and commit all kinds of silly, foolish acts. One patient, who had succeeded with difficulty in becoming a school teacher, suddenly became completely incapable of doing his job, could not run his class, played tig with the children instead of teaching them, lay down in a manger in the cowshed 'just for fun' and stuck his head into the fountain because he needed to be re-baptised because of his great sins. A striking feature in such behaviour is frequent affectless laughter, which is repeated during every interview and for which there is not the slightest reason. It is not based on levity of mood; on the contrary, patients sometimes report that it comes over them irresistibly, against their will. Occasionally they also exhibit grimacing, grunting, stereotyped postures and movements, or elaborate and affected gestures.

Their speech contains theatrical declamations, repetition of certain mannerisms, stale jokes, high-sounding phrases, deliberate distortion of words, affecting lisping, and the use of unusual expressions, phrases or sentences, perhaps in dialect or foreign languages. Many of the same characteristics appear even more plainly in the patients' writings. Here we find careless and incoherent thinking, long drawn out sentences with many changes of construction, a mixture of different kinds of imagery, the sudden introduction of new ideas and rhymed effusions that are often like a sort of song. The writing is asymmetrical, individual letters are disfigured by flourishes and underlinings, and there are either too few or too many punctuation marks. In fact, the patients' letters are often so characteristic that on the basis of them alone it is possible to make an assured diagnosis of this special form of mental impairment.

The course of the illness varies, in that the dementia may proceed at a slow or fast rate, or be halted at different stages. In the most favourable cases the illness ends after a few months or years in a state of severe mental impairment. The condition then remains unaltered for the rest of the patient's life, though at times it would seem that some of the symptoms gradually disappear. The premorbid level of mental ability is never fully regained. There are probably many people who have suffered a mental breakdown due to dementia praecox, but who have never been diagnosed as such because they have managed to retain sufficient mental ability to survive the struggle for existence and to pursue modest activities. Many industrious and even gifted pupils may belong to this category; they start off with justifiably high hopes, but later, and in spite of effort and conscientious striving, disappoint their teachers and have the greatest difficulty in attaining what their far less-talented classmates achieve with ease. Of course, only precise knowledge and follow-up of individual cases can provide proof of morbid change. Because of their incapacity for regular work, such mentally crippled youngsters often join the ranks of beggars and vagrants, perhaps later to be admitted to the work-house or the asylum. In other cases we find that after a few years the degree of mental impairment is such that they can no longer live independent lives, though within the framework of an institution or in family care a certain measure of mental or practical activity can be maintained.

The patients who come to the attention of the psychiatrist are not as a rule those with the milder forms of illness described above. In the large majority of cases the clinical picture is much more stormy. The illness in these cases often begins gradually. The early signs are headache, buzzing in the ears, confusion, giddiness, tiredness, and surly, irritable, withdrawn behaviour. The patient sleeps badly, loses his appetite, becomes run down physically and seems to be inert and apathetic, slovenly and forgetful, and either does not pursue his usual activities at all or performs them badly with many interruptions. His mood is now nearly always depressed, with self-reproach, groundless weeping, thoughts of death, and sometimes even sudden and unexpected suicidal attempts. He has given false testimony, indulged in self-abuse, fallen into evil ways, is damned beyond hope of redemption. No one can help him, everything has gone wrong for him and his life is worth nothing. He may busy himself night and day with religious texts and express a wish to enter a monastery.

At the same time he has all kinds of vague ideas of persecution. He becomes suspicious of those around him, sees poison in his food, is pursued by the police, feels his body is being influenced, or thinks that he is going to be shot or that the neighbours are jeering at him. He may, however, feel very definitely that he is ill: he feels he is not free, his head is not clear, he is no longer as he used to be; reason, understanding and sense have fled from his brain. At times such ideas assume a hypochondriacal form. Something has got into his head, his blood is not circulating, his stomach is not functioning, his insides are burned up and rotten. I have seen two such patients, whose hypochondriacal ideas fitted in with earlier ailments from which they thought they had not yet recovered.

Hallucinations are also common, especially auditory experiences of abuse, threats, demands, whispers, which in some circumstances seem to influence the patient's actions. It is not usually possible to learn more from the patient about these subjective experiences. As a rule he says little, is timid or preoccupied, and at times even confused and unintelligible. His mood at this stage is usually depressed or anxious. Often, however, there is a marked degree of apathy and indifference, which bears no relation to the content of his delusional ideas and hallucinations. The patient may often laugh unexpectedly and with no good reason; at times he may show angry or anxious irritability, with violent emotional outbursts.

The most striking feature, however, is the lack of inner consistency in his speech and behaviour. He gives meaningless, incoherent, disjointed answers, and talks at times foolishly in incomprehensible sentences. He suddenly goes bathing with his clothes on, kisses the ground, makes a childish attempt at suicide, attacks members of his family, undresses in the street, wanders off aimlessly for weeks at a time, and when reproached offers the vaguest reasons for his behaviour. Often it is this kind of extraordinary and senseless behaviour that first makes his relatives aware of the developing mental disturbance. A postman, who had hitherto carried out his duties without interruption, one day signed an official document as Field Marshal General, demanded a helmet and the uniform of a general, said he was the son of Kaiser Wilhelm and that he knew from his supervisor's fingernails that he was his brother.

As the delusional ideas disappear and the affective symptoms fade this first stage of the illness may, within a few months or years, imperceptibly, and with no intermediate episodes, pass into simple dementia. In many cases, however, there are outbursts of florid, expansive excitement, sometimes accompanied by sudden mood swings and in women often coinciding with menstruation. The patients become merry, carefree and talkative; they relate all kinds of fabricated experiences, and express confused, not always very magnificent, ideas of grandeur: they have a lot of money, a room full of gold, beautiful clothes, they want to go and see the Emperor, join the Army, become a parson, an actress. They are at the same time poorly oriented towards their environment; although they recognise individual persons, they do not know precisely where they are or what is happening to them, and they are incapable of assessing their situation.

As a rule these phenomena are accompanied by a state of lively sexual excitement. They claim to have been married for fifty years; they have had twenty-two wives; they want a girl, demand sexual intercourse, masturbate. There is not usually much motor unrest. Loud, incessant talking and shouting are exceptional and occur only when nursing care is inadequate, as does beating on doors, unclean behaviour, tearing of clothes and undressing. Left to themselves, the patients are inclined to run away and go wandering; they soon come to grief, commit silly, senseless acts or sexual excesses and usually come very quickly into conflict with the law. In individual cases their state may closely resemble one of hysterical excitement. The similarity becomes even greater if, as sometimes happens, there are accompanying fainting fits, ocular gyrations, fits of laughing, dyspnoea and convulsive attacks.

The expansive excitement, which rarely manifests itself in the form of ideas of grandeur, the euphoric mood and the groundless laughter do not usually persist for long in pronounced form. After a few months or less, the symptoms fade and the condition appears to have improved. But, although the patients become calmer, it is at this point that signs of severe mental impairment begin to emerge. Usually this develops into a simple, apathetic dementia, though occasionally a certain degree of cheerful, silly excitement will be maintained, even in states of advanced dementia, a feature more characteristic of women than of men.

In patients with transient but clear-cut delusions, the illness follows a different course. In the early stages, ideas of persecution predominate, associated with ideas of bodily influence. The patient finds poison in his food, 'hobnail juice and potash', feels contractions in his spinal cord, hears voices in his genitals, and thinks he is two people. He is being anaesthetised, bewitched, blinded with mirrors, denounced as a spy, will be sentenced to eternal damnation. He is being debauched, his semen has been removed. Female patients often complain of sexual assault. Other people read their thoughts, imitate their actions, suggest words to them. They hear voices which repeat everything they say, urge them to commit suicide. They see the devil sitting before them; they are fit only to be executed; they will never be healthy again.

At a later stage ideas of grandeur often gain the upper hand. The patient has come into a huge inheritance, he is descended from the Kaiser, he has lived in the world for thousands of years, he sees visions of the saints in heaven, he converses with God. At night he has intercourse with the Holy Spirit. Dream experiences are often turned into delusions, or into a fabricated adventure. The patient has been to Paradise, he comes from the land of Job, he was an army doctor hundreds of years ago in America, he thinks he is 'the Northern Lights', or 'Mount Horeb'. As a rule, such absurdities have a florid onset and then fade into the background: they become more meagre and finally disappear altogether, or persist only as a few isolated, incoherent, fragmentary ideas which crop up at rare intervals in response to explicit questions or in moments of excitement. At the same time the initial high spirits or irritable mood changes to apathy and indifference.

It would seem that in most cases the disease progresses into a state of profound dementia. The patients sink lower and lower, and become silly and apathetic, losing all understanding of their surroundings. Often their eating habits deteriorate, they gulp greedily and smear their food around them; they soil themselves, retain faeces and urine, dribble spittle over their clothes. Their voluntary movements may cease; they stand or sit wherever they happen to find themselves, mute and idle; they make occasional silly comments; they have to be dressed and undressed, fed and moved about.

In response to external stimuli, they may be passive, cataleptic or resistant. Their sparse answers are usually quite irrelevant, showing only occasionally some understanding of the question; simple but firm requests are sometimes correctly obeyed, and a few individuals known to them from their past are correctly named. They succeed now and again in displaying remnants of knowledge from their schooldays – correct reading or writing, the right answer to a sum, or the retention of some historical, geographical or grammatical fact. In time, however, such traces of earlier mental functioning gradually disappear, until finally only an isolated, very firmly-rooted memory bears witness to the fact that what we have here is not uncultivated or barren ground but land that has been laid waste. Sometimes clear traces remain of the earlier excited state, with confused, incomprehensible sentences, foolish laughter, affected movements and expressions, and violent rushing up and down. Often the patients show transient phases of irritation: they will suddenly rush outside, use bad language, act violently, break a window pane, throw a key to the ground, tear one of their garments or strike an unexpected blow at a room-mate. They may pluck at their clothes, tie them in knots, drape themselves dramatically in their garments, pluck hair from their beard or head, scratch themselves persistently in certain parts of the body and openly masturbate.

In my experience the development of dementia praecox is usually accompanied by a series of bodily disturbances. Apart from the changes in sleep and appetite which also occur in states of excitement and affective disorders, some symptoms which point to an increase in nervous excitability deserve particular mention. The tendon reflexes are very often lively and in many cases there is an increase in muscular reactivity and skin responses. Menstruation is often irregular or ceases entirely. In two cases the illness was preceded by a pronounced attack of tetany. Finally, in a number of cases fainting fits occurred in the course of the illness. I recently saw a slightly older student. From adolescence he had been particularly gifted but suddenly fell into a deep coma from which he only very gradually awakened. Apart from slight pupillary change, facial symptoms and increased reflex activity, there was no evidence of cerebral damage. When I examined him a few weeks later, however, he presented a clear picture of premature mental impairment.

The course of dementia praecox is generally regular and progressive.

It is rare to see a substantial remission of the symptoms; at least the excitement disappears, but the mental impairment remains. On the other hand, it is fairly common to find patients who are calm, whose condition has 'improved', but who revert even after years to a state of excitement. Body weight usually decreases steadily in the early stages and when the patient is excited. As he begins to calm down and dementia sets in, the body weight rises again, often considerably, so that patients begin to look positively blooming as their appetite increases.

The most common outcome in severe forms of dementia praecox is dementia. In many cases the patients' outward bearing may remain fairly intact after the more stormy symptoms have subsided. They are fairly well oriented as to their surroundings and situation; they show some insight into the illness they have suffered; but at the same time they can keep going only if their lives follow the most simple pattern. They take no part in what goes on around them, and show no interest in the passage of time or in their means of subsistence, though with precise instructions they are often able to make themselves useful in small ways. Apart from the intellectual defect, the most common residual symptoms of the illness are irritability, sensitivity to alcohol, occasional states of excitement, odd modes of expression and peculiar behavioural habits.

We should also include here those isolated cases in which the delusions and hallucinations of the excited phase gradually fade into the background but are still liable to recur transiently from time to time. Occasionally we find persistent hallucinations which do not seem to affect the patient and which they rarely mention. Sometimes, however, particularly during menstruation, such patients may suddenly become excited, with vivid hallucinations, persecutory and grandiose ideas, and destructive urges. After a short time they calm down and regain insight into their condition. One cannot talk about persistent, firm delusions in such cases. It is more a question of weakness of judgement.

After the illness has run its course there is no real possibility of further educational pursuits; at best, one can expect to maintain the patient's condition in some degree of stability. It is relatively rare for the patient to be able to return to even a modest degree of mental independence.

Dementia praecox is a very common illness. During the last five years it has accounted for five to six per cent of admissions to my clinic. Very little is known at present of the causes of the disorder. We do know, however, that it is particularly liable to develop in adolescence and early childhood. In more than half the cases I have collected, the onset was between the ages of 16 and 22. Further experience may, of course, reveal cases with a later onset, which today are given a different diagnosis. It is certain, however, that the large majority of cases of sudden onset and eventual dementia belong to the younger age groups. For this reason dementia praecox has in the past been called 'youthful insanity' or 'hebephrenia'. Men appear to be three times more likely than women to suffer from the forms of illness described here, a fact which seems strange when one considers the reverse ratio in catatonia. An inherited predisposition occurred in about 70 per cent of the cases which were closely scrutinised, and so-called signs of degeneracy were often observed: smallness or deformity of the skull, child-like habitus, missing teeth, deformed ears. The patient's original abilities had usually been good, often better than average; occasionally, however, some degree of mental debility had been evident from early age. A number of my patients showed a diffuse enlargement of the thyroid. I cannot, however, attach any special significance to this finding, in view of the great frequency of the same phenomenon in this neighbourhood.

The first precise, and in many respects exemplary, description of certain forms of dementia praecox was given by Hecker in 1871. He was influenced by Kahlbaum's description of certain cases of mental disorder and observed that melancholia followed by mania often turned into a quite specific form of mental debility. Only a small proportion of the cases which I regard as dementia praecox would fall into the category of hebephrenia in this sense. Daraszkiewicz, in his dissertation of 1892, extended the concept of hebephrenia to cover the severe forms which end in profound dementia. I believe that provisionally we should retain the term dementia praecox for the extended group of illnesses.

As Hecker pointed out, the age of onset is usually adolescence or early adulthood. It is this which lends a distinctive stamp to the mental disability that constitutes the end stage of hebephrenia. Hecker was inclined to think that the outcome of his hebephrenia represented an arrest of all psychic life at the developmental stage of puberty. Against this argument is the fact that a large number of cases of severe debility show a regression and not just an arrest of mental development. In premature dementia we still find many features which we recognise easily from healthy developmental stages. For example, there is the inclination to read inappropriate material, the naive preoccupation with lofty problems, an immature and over-ready speed of judgement, and a delight in catch-words and high-sounding modes of speech . . .

The real nature of dementia praecox is totally obscure. The most common view at present is that the illness occurs when an individual's inadequate constitutional faculties gradually cease to function. Like a tree whose roots no longer find nourishment in the earth available to it, mental powers dwindle as soon as an insufficient natural endowment makes further development impossible. There are, however, serious objections to this point of view. It is hard to see why an organism which has hitherto developed in a healthy or even energetic way should suddenly, and for no particular reason, not only come to a standstill but even deteriorate into chronic sickness. Even the most severely morbid predisposition – which is not particularly common in dementia praecox anyway – would hardly suffice to explain such a process. Moreover, those mental disorders which are known to be associated with hereditary degeneration do not show this kind of sudden mental deterioration: in such cases periodic illnesses or persistent morbid states with a very slow development are more common.

For these reasons I consider it more likely that what we have here is a tangible morbid process occurring in the brain. Only in this way does the quick descent into severe dementia become at all comprehensible. It is true that morbid anatomy has so far been quite unable to help us here, but we should not forget that reliable methods have not yet been employed in a serious search for morbid changes. In the light of our current experience, I would assume that we are dealing here with an auto-intoxication, whose immediate causes lie somewhere in the body. This assumption seems to me to be supported by the appearance of fairly significant physical signs in the nerves and muscles of patients with dementia praecox. If we consider the tendency for the illness to strike at the age when sexual development is still taking place, then it is not out of the question for there to be a connection between the illness and some processes taking place in the sexual organs. These are, of course, only provisional and very indefinite hypotheses.

It is of the greatest practical importance to diagnose cases of dementia praecox with certainty and at an early stage. The main differential diagnoses are periodic insanity [manic-depressive psychosis, Tr.], paranoia and organic psychosis due to a recognisable physical illness. The features which suggest dementia praecox rather than periodic insanity are a slow onset, less intense symptoms, and signs of acquired mental debility. Against paranoia are a rapid development, the scant and confused nature of such delusional ideas as are present, and the growing mental impairment that very soon becomes apparent. In our current concept of paranoia, however, there are transitional forms, which we may possibly come to recognise as special types of the dementing process. In favour of a typical organic psychosis would be an acute impairment of all mental functions, a sudden onset and the accompanying physical signs. In addition, many cases of dementia praecox are wrongly diagnosed as mental subnormality. In view of the great prognostic difference between these two disorders, such mistakes exact a bitter toll. It is very difficult to differentiate between dementia praecox and innate imbecility. I have had several patients with apparent severe mental deficiency, brought to me from the workhouse with convictions for begging, vagrancy and similar offences, who were incapable of giving even the most meagre information about their past lives. It was later possible to demonstrate, however, that they had some vestiges of passable scholastic attainment; in one case, for example, letters were obtained which showed that the patient, who was not a complete imbecile, had a few years earlier been able to travel in a planned way and to express his thoughts with fluency and skill. It was clear, therefore, that it was not a question of mental subnormality, but of acquired dementia praecox. Such cases are of particular interest to military physicians, as symptoms of illness frequently appear just before or during military service and may then easily be mistaken for deliberate simulation.

Given our present ignorance of the causes of the illness, the treatment of dementia praecox offers few points for intervention. One may perhaps assume, however, that timely safeguards against aggravating the cerebral condition, combined with treatment of sleeplessness, excitement and refusal of food, may halt the mental deterioration at a certain stage, and this may facilitate the use of what has not yet been destroyed. Once the acute stage of the illness is quiescent, it becomes a question of instituting cautious mental exercise of such abilities as are still present, in order to protect these residual abilities from the atrophy that may take place if they are not used.

Reference

Hecker, E. (1871) Die Hebephrenie. *Virchows Archiv für pathologische Anatomie* **52**, 392–449.

Otto Diem (circa 1895–)

Otto Diem was born in Switzerland, where he spent his whole professional life. He trained under Eugen Bleuler at the Burghölzli Clinic in Zurich and then devoted himself to clinical psychiatry in Lucerne.

His article on simple schizophrenia or dementia simplex was probably suggested by Eugen Bleuler and was an elaboration of an earlier idea of Arnold Pick's. Nevertheless, it is one of the few clinical studies in the literature of a condition which, although controversial, has become part of established psychiatric nosology.

The simple dementing form of dementia praecox

O. Diem (1903)

(Die einfach demente Form der Dementia praecox. *Archiv für Psychiatrie und Nervenkrankheiten* **37**, 111–87)

Case histories

The following cases are presented to illustrate the argument of this paper.

Case 1

The patient was a lively boy, with no particular behavioural problems. He successfully attended state school, then technical school and finally completed a three-year apprenticeship as a photographer. He took part in the campaigns of 1866 and 1870 as a non-commissioned officer in the German army. Then he began work as a photographer but drifted around restlessly as an assistant or journeyman, never staying longer than three years in one place. He changed jobs in order to 'see something new', never because of disagreement with his employers. Two attempts to set him up in business on his own account failed miserably. He lost all his money, evidently because he took too little trouble and was too lighthearted in his approach to the undertaking. He married during this period, at the age of about forty, but his wife died a few years later; the marriage was apparently a happy one. He then left his parents-in-law to look after his children and thereafter did not bother about them in the slightest. From then on he never prospered, although he was active in all kinds of affairs, sometimes on his own account, sometimes as a journeyman or just as a messenger. He often sat around in inns, but was not a heavy drinker. No special information is available about his sexual life. For about six months he was indifferent to everything, slept a lot, sat all day in his room, read newspapers, and took no interest in his children or other relatives. Once he lay in bed for four weeks, doing nothing. He told careless and obvious lies.

An old rheumatic complaint in his joints flared up again and he had to spend a long time in hospital, from which he was transferred to an institution, because 'he had no energy, had sunk into a low moral state, his intellectual capacity was reduced, and he was unable to maintain himself or to do anything useful'. The initial diagnosis on admission was primary dementia . . .

On admission and throughout his hospital stay he showed no interest in his own condition or in the external world. He did not know, for example, whether his three children were still alive. He spoke in a quiet manner about what had happened to him, attributing everything to his physical illness. He remembered the past well, and was quick at arithmetic, but was only moderately well informed geographically and had only the roughest idea about recent political events. On physical examination he was normal except for a fine tremor of the hands. Although he had been a moderate drinker in the past, he was virtually abstinent during the years of his admission and the argument against a diagnosis of alcoholic dementia rests on his previous history, the observation that he does not now indulge in alcohol and the fact that his condition has shown no improvement during his stay. There were no delusions, no hallucinations and no mannerisms or negativism.

Case 2

The second patient was a man, aged 62 when admitted to hospital.

As a boy he had done well at school and the local priest had encouraged him to study theology. His mother was against this and so he remained at home helping her with her silk weaving. At the age of 18 he quarrelled with his parents, and was so aggrieved that he considered throwing himself in the river. Instead he joined up as a mercenary in a Swiss regiment. He served for seven years, which he later regarded as the best years of his life. He could have become a non-commissioned officer but preferred to stay in the ranks. After this he returned home to work as a weaver with his mother. He married at the age of 28 but did not get on well with his wife and from time to time lived apart from her because she was lazy and extravagant and frittered away all his money. They were divorced 11 years later. He moved from place to place, working in various factories and never staying anywhere for long.

During his 50s he was frequently under the care of the local authorities, because he hardly ever worked; he caused trouble about the food, was abusive and often lay in bed out of sheer laziness. He had been travelling around as a pedlar and drinking heavily.

On admission to hospital a provisional diagnosis of dementia, possibly alcoholic in origin, was made . . .

During his six-year stay in hospital his mental state remained unchanged. His physical state was normal apart from a fine tremor of the hands. He was invariably cheerful, had a good memory, and conversed and played cards with other patients. He was well orientated and was quick with calculations. He held his mother responsible for thwarting his ambition to do better in life and blamed the local authorities for having placed him in the hospital but, now he was a patient here, he said he felt quite content. He had no delusions and no hallucinations. He had an affected manner of speaking, with frequent moralising and hectoring, but had no mannerisms or negativistic features.

Discussion

Clinical features

Although there is a wide variation in the way in which this condition presents itself, common to all cases is the onset of a change in mental state soon after puberty. This occurs gradually: an individual becomes unstable, lacking in willpower and self-control, and wanders around aimlessly, often finishing up after a period of vagrancy in his home district. In many cases there is an unmistakable decline in performance, a narrowing of mental horizons and a restriction of thinking; they cannot carry out their former jobs adequately and have to be replaced because their work is unsatisfactory. A change in personality takes place, the most prominent feature of which is that an individual becomes more excitable and quarrelsome, often lascivious, and is never content, but finds something to criticise in everything. He never sees himself as in the wrong, but considers himself misunderstood, oppressed and downtrodden. He may say that he is 'persecuted', but this never reaches the stage of a genuine delusion of persecution. It never occurs to him that he might himself be to blame and rejects any such idea absolutely and indignantly.

As a result of these mental changes, an individual may begin to drink heavily. Some, who have quarrelled with their relatives, sign on for service abroad or for other reasons move to distant countries, to America and Australia. On their return after a few years they are penniless and show no inclination to organise themselves or to work. Many are regularly sent back by the authorities to their home district, where they cannot be kept for long in private houses because of their difficult behaviour and marked avoidance of work. Eventually, when no one will take them in, they are sent to an institution.

In the institution they are usually quiet, with an impoverishment of affect which contrasts with their previous reported agitation. This change in their emotional state can be attributed to the discipline and the general atmosphere of the institution, and also to their abstinence from alcohol. It is true that almost all the patients are excitable and at times turbulent if something vexes them; they are violent over trifles and sometimes abuse the authorities who have had them admitted. Many, however, who were said to have behaved previously in this manner, become much quieter. All show, for most of the time, a mood of indifference; they go their ways quietly, many sit still and inactive, each after his fashion. Some say that they are sad, though there are no visible signs of a marked depression. The level of activity of these patients is significantly reduced and one never encounters a lively or even a moderate pressure of activity. The patients are capable of sitting around all day quite happily without doing anything and without becoming bored. Some patients are persuaded by the conduct of those around them or by special inducements, such as additional money, tobacco or permission to go out, to join in the institution's activities. They then help with the work but do it mechanically, without taking time for consideration and without showing any of the mental alertness that takes account of the varying circumstances involved in a job of work. It was just this lack of alertness, of adaptability, that had made these individuals fail in their own social level earlier in their lives.

The awareness of the patients suffers to a similar degree. They still take in the ordinary daily events of the institution, but they do no more than register them; there is no question of their taking a lively interest in what is happening and is going to happen. They accept all external events with indifference so long as they are not directly and adversely affected, when they quickly become excited. They are also indifferent to their families, relatives and friends; on the whole they write few and not very cordial letters and when visitors come they receive them coldly and listlessly, making little effort to renew relationships or to keep up appearances. But their apathy is most clearly demonstrated by the almost stoical way in which they accept their lot and in which they are able to listen while people harangue them about what they have missed in life and the seriousness of their present situation in regard to their career and its downward trend. A slight, conventional expression of regret is the most that one can achieve in the way of response . . .

A number of patients show a characteristic mode of thinking, though it is not easy to say precisely what this is. In talking to them one is struck by the way in which, while apparently following the thread of the conversation and expressing a given thought quite correctly, they will often switch to another subject which has no recognisable connection with what was being said. It is as if they had plucked a new topic out of the air, which they then introduce with some irrelevant phrase such as 'It's just like . . .', 'I have also thought. . .' or 'People say . . .'. It is not difficult to bring the conversation back to the original subject by asking a suitably related question. The patients themselves do not seem to be aware of their digression, which might be called a 'side-slip'. This type of disturbance is akin to the phenomenon often encountered in florid dementia praecox, where word associations are formed with completely unrelated words, giving the impression that they are genuine ideas. The disturbance has been variously described as 'disconnectedness', 'thought distraction' or 'incoherence in the flow of ideas', but perhaps the term 'interruption in the flow of ideas' best conveys the essential nature of the phenomenon. Another frequently encountered symptom is for a patient's answers, while not directly irrelevant, to be very imprecise, not to the point and somewhat inappropriate. Some authors have attributed this to a general disturbance of attention, though this cannot adequately account for the ideational leaps which were mentioned above . . .

There is some similarity between the condition described here and Bonnhoeffer's description of patients who are moderately defective from birth and who shortly before puberty begin to live a very antisocial life, with a tendency to heavy drinking, restless vagrancy, frequent criminal activity and rejection of discipline even in an institution. Cramer also referred to similar cases with mental debility developing around puberty, accompanied by behaviour which led to conflict with the law.

Aetiology
A family history of mental illness was present in 15 out of the 19 cases of this condition that I have studied. In eight of these at least one parent

had been clearly mentally ill. In the remaining seven cases a more distant relative had been affected or a parent was described as 'peculiar' or eccentric . . .

It is not possible to comment on any pathological changes in the brain, because the brains of two of the 19 patients who died were not available to us . . .

The upbringing in some patients was unfavourable, but in others it was exemplary, and so this factor cannot be regarded as particularly relevant . . .

The case-histories were incomplete with respect to previous physical illnesses, and the importance of this factor too must remain uncertain . . .

Even the relevance of puberty must be in question, because several patients developed their first symptoms in their twenties . . .

Course of illness

The illness began insidiously and progressed by degrees to an end state characterised by moderately severe feeblemindedness, after which it would remain stable. The excitability tended to diminish, but genuine remissions of the actual illness were unknown. There was no recovery: the patients learned to adapt to the ways of the institution and became automatic in their behaviour. The mental debility persisted, but it cannot be said that the illness became recognisably worse. In time the patients became somewhat more apathetic, but this is a fate which they share with all other inmates of large institutions where the regime is uniform and unchangeable.

Retrospectively, of course, we were usually unable to get more than an approximate idea of the age at which the first signs of illness appeared. The information recorded on admission was often, for good reasons, inadequate in this respect, the onset in all cases being so gradual that no one could say definitely when the illness had begun. Nevertheless in most cases it was possible to arrive at some point of reference. According to this kind of assessment the age of onset could be said to lie approximately between the ages of 15 and 50. In eight cases it was between 15 and 22, and in seven between 25 and 30. In the two cases in which our information pointed to a later onset, the early history was very inadequate and it was possible that the illness had begun much earlier.

Admission to an institution took place because the patients were without means, so that it was a last resort on the part of the authorities. The patients were nearly always admitted a considerable time after onset of the illness, this ranging from a minimum of one year to a maximum of 44 years (Case 2 above). In most instances it was about 25 to 35 years after the illness had begun.

Prior to admission patients had been dealt with as the need arose. It was not that they lived in peace and quiet – on the contrary, they had for years or decades been a cross which their families, their relatives, the authorities and the police had had to bear. Most of them had for years been a burden on the community. Not only had others to be responsible for their upkeep, since they did no work or could not be relied upon to work, but most of them were unpleasant in character, being so quarrelsome and full of complaints that people were genuinely glad to have them admitted somewhere even if it meant paying for them. Many, however, removed themselves from the care of the authorities and wandered restlessly around from one place to another, mostly ending up without means in their home district . . .

When hitherto amenable wives and mothers gradually become quarrelsome and cantankerous, when they can no longer accept the slightest contradiction, when they are cold to their husbands and reject them and when they live in discord with everybody, the effect on family life is devastating. At times it seems as if one is dealing with a depraved character, though in the end the contumacy and hopelessness of the condition leads to the conviction that the person is not wicked but sick. Often, however, it is the professional verdict of the doctor that first conveys this information to the family, since the absence of symptoms that are usually associated with mental illness prevents the layman from reaching such a conclusion. It is not hard to appreciate how much time is usually spent in disagreeable family quarrels, misunderstandings and vexations before the patience and forbearance of the tormented relatives are at an end, and they seek professional advice. It will be appreciated, therefore, how important it is to be familiar with the course of the illness, so that its diagnosis can be correctly made at an early stage. Much bitterness and family distress will then be avoided. It is a similar story with the poor law authorities and officials of charitable institutions, who may believe they are dealing with straightforward disorderly, rootless people, vagrants and drunkards, and therefore approach them via a disciplinary regime. Early recognition of the deeper disturbance would save much useless effort . . .

Diagnosis and differential diagnosis

The end state in this condition may differ in degree, but in kind it is always the same: a moderate degree of mental debility, dullness and apathy with moments of excitability, a loss of mental alertness, an inability to act independently and a marked lack of judgement; at the same time comprehension and orientation are maintained and memory is not noticeably affected. These are precisely the characteristics of that special form of mental debility found in Hecker's hebephrenia and in Kraepelin's dementia praecox. This would seem to confirm the proposal to place the condition alongside other types of dementia praecox, and this is further strengthened by the existence of transitional forms amongst my 19 cases. My reason for wishing to separate these cases from the general group of dementia praecox, and to designate them as the simple dementing form of that illness, is the importance of recognising its particular course. It deserves to be given a special position, since acute symptoms are lacking and if there is any ambiguity the insidious dementing process which presents itself to the psychiatrist may be mistaken for simulation or hostile inactivity.

Pure cases of this condition are not common, but this is also true of the other forms of dementia praecox. We know that hebephrenia, catatonia and dementia paranoides can pass imperceptibly one into another . . .

On the question of differential diagnosis, individual cases are often mistaken for alcoholic dementia. In the latter condition, however, one would expect the dementia to improve with abstinence and, even if we accept the existence of a pure and irreversible alcoholic dementia, there would have had to be a different pattern and longer duration of excessive drinking. Furthermore, the end state of our patients is quite different from the mental state found in chronic alcoholics. The latter, in particular, tend to be emotionally labile, and make foolish and frantic attempts to leave hospital in order to obtain alcohol.

General paralysis can be excluded because of the absence of any physical symptoms, the often excellent memory and the course of the illness. Cerebral disorders due to such causes as tumours, trauma, multiple sclerosis and focal syphilitic lesions can also be dismissed as an explanation in the cases I have reported: the period of observation was too long for there to be any doubt about this point.

In several of the cases in my series hysteria might be an alternative diagnosis. But if this were so, one would expect an entirely different course, marked by fluctuations and emotional outbursts.

Two of the 19 cases had been diagnosed elsewhere as paranoia. A careful analysis of the patients' mental state would have shown how incorrect this diagnosis was. The two patients believed that they were underestimated and even scorned but never entertained the notion that any action against them was deliberate and logical. In both cases the alleged paranoia was only loosely associated with the characteristic dementia.

Senile and other organic dementias can be excluded because of the lack of any clear disturbances of memory and attention. There was also none of the characteristic emotional incontinence and no intermittent disturbances of consciousness.

Neurasthenia need not be considered seriously since the patients' previous history and the course of their illness leave no doubt on this score. There are, however, some isolated nervous symptoms common to both disorders, so that in the initial stages the differential diagnosis may present some difficulties.

Summary

In addition to the clinical pictures presented by hebephrenia, catatonia and dementia paranoides, the end state of all these being the characteristic mental debility of Kraepelin's dementia praecox, there is one further condition which leads to the same end state, to the same disorder of intelligence and affect. The onset of this particular form of the illness is habitually simple, insidious and without warning signs, and the illness develops without acute progressive attacks and remissions. There are no definite affective disturbances of a manic or melancholic nature, no hallucinations or delusional ideas, and none of the characteristic symptoms of the other forms of dementia praecox which I have just listed, such as catalepsy, affectations, mannerisms, stereotypies, negativism and mutism.

After some years the illness usually reaches a fairly stable state. By analogy with the simple dementing form of general paralysis it seems best to introduce this type of course into the literature as the simple dementing form of dementia praecox, or true dementia simplex, and to continue to use this term from now on.

Pure cases of this form of dementia praecox are not very common, but may be more common than is realised, since they are seen professionally only very briefly or come under detailed observation only at a very late stage when they are admitted to institutions. What has been classified by Kahlbaum and Weygandt as heboidophrenia and by Sommer and others as primary dementia refers almost entirely to transitional forms of hebephrenia. There are no adequate grounds for treating such forms as a separate entity since they share not only the same course and outcome as hebephrenia but also the same chief symptoms. They cannot be differentiated on the basis of the type of phenomena, but only by their severity. In this they resemble two of the cases in this series, which demonstrate the possibility of transitional stages between the simple dementing and the hebephrenic subtypes. Twelve of our cases, however, showed no specifically hebephrenic symptoms whatsoever, either on admission or during the entire course of the illness, which justifies our designating them as a separate and clearly delimited diagnostic category, either as pure cases under the rubric of the simple dementing form of dementia praecox, or as true dementia simplex.

This strict categorisation is, however, somewhat artificial. Mood swings, catatonic symptoms or delusional ideas may arise, and lead to the most varied and transitional forms of dementia praecox as has already been described. Borderline cases of hebephrenia are the most common, but there may also be borderline cases of catatonia and dementia paranoides. There are also fleeting transitions to the querulant forms of dementia praecox. Women are very often wrongly diagnosed as 'bad characters', men as alcoholics.

A symptom of dementia praecox that receives little mention, but which was frequently found in our material, is a fine, fairly regular tremor of the hands.

In the present state of our knowledge it is not possible in the early stages of the illness to predict what the course is likely to be. Even after years the clinical picture may change. For example, an illness which has been following the course of a simple dementia may shift into the hebephrenic form.

The simple dementing, hebephrenic and catatonic forms of dementia praecox form clinically one unitary psychosis.

The aetiology of the illness requires more thorough study. Neither puberty nor heredity is sufficient to account for its occurrence.

The simple dementing form of dementia praecox is of great practical and forensic significance and deserves the consideration of the medical practitioner, particularly in view of its close relationship with alcoholism, vagrancy and acquired personality disorder.

Otto Gross (1877–1920)

Otto Gross was born in Graz in Austria and died in Berlin at the age of 33. He was an eccentric person, an alcoholic and a drug addict who consulted Freud, Jung and Gruhle. Jung regarded him as schizophrenic. He was an anarchist in the years before the First World War, took part in the socialist revolutions which convulsed Germany and Austria after the war, and was friendly with Max Brod and Franz Kafka in Prague.

Despite his own psychiatric illness, he wrote extensively and sensibly on a variety of aspects of organic and functional psychoses. The following extract is a comment on the idea, current at the time, that schizophrenia was a disorder of consciousness.

Dementia sejunctiva
O. Gross (1904)
(*Neurologisches Centralblatt* **23**, 1144–6)

In a previous paper I proposed that the term 'dementia sejunctiva' be introduced to replace the term 'dementia praecox'. Stransky has since criticised my proposal, and the purpose of the present paper is to present my own counter arguments.

The meaning of the term 'dementia' has changed in current psychiatric usage. We have grown accustomed to employing it to denote not only an end state but also a developing state, a process. As the term is used today, therefore, we have to understand it, according to circumstances, sometimes as 'imbecility' or 'feeblemindedness' and sometimes as 'becoming imbecilic', 'dementing'. When Kraepelin established this terminology he gave the name 'dementia' to certain clinical pictures and described them collectively as 'processes of dementing'. I have retained this usage and would like the word 'dementia' to be understood in my proposed nomenclature as a 'process of dementing' in the widest sense.

In designating clinical illnesses one usually tries to find a name which implies an aetiology or, if this is not possible, a name which indicates a markedly conspicuous symptom.

Sejunction is a universal and cardinal psychopathological symptom that occurs prominently in most acute psychoses, far more so in fact than in chronic or subacute phases or forms of the dementia praecox group of illnesses. 'Dementia sejunctiva', however, is a double-barrel-led term and means that the factor of sejunction is regarded as particularly conspicuous in one group only among the many forms of dementia. This means only that sejunction has more significance for the dementia praecox group than for the other groups of illnesses that we call the 'dementias'. I would also claim not only that sejunction plays a greater part in dementia praecox than in all the other dementing processes, but also that it is the most striking and dominant of all the phenomena of that condition. In other words, the symptomatology of dementia praecox, in contrast to all other forms of dementia, is dominated by sejunction.

Sejunction, in my sense, means a breakdown of consciousness of a particular type. It is the simultaneous collapse of several functionally separate series of associations. The most important component of the concept is that the activity of consciousness always has to be seen as the product of many simultaneously ongoing psychophysical proces-ses. The unity of consciousness is never apparent to us in its entirety, but is produced by the synthesis of simultaneous processes. This synthesising activity can be suspended by functional disturbances of an unknown kind, and that is what I mean by the sejunction mechanism.

My views on sejunction were derived from those of Wernicke, but there are some differences in our two concepts, which I should like to emphasise. Wernicke treats the activity of consciousness as a succes-sion of events in time, never as the co-existence and intertwining of simultaneous processes, as I do. Whereas in Wernicke's scheme, the sejunction mechanism is a 'closed circuit' of associative ties, in mine it is the work of synthesis which is affected. Wernicke's explanation of sejunction involves the loss of certain associations caused by an interruption in pathways. I invoke a general decline in some higher cerebral function. Wernicke's sejunction factors are theoretically localisable, whereas mine are diffuse. In summary, Wernicke is more concerned with a breakdown in the contents of consciousness, whereas my formulation emphasises the process involved.

When Stransky made his own valuable contribution to the under-standing of dementia praecox, in which he emphasised the 'striking disparity between affective and intellectual life', he maintained that such dissociation was incompatible with Wernicke's concept of sejunc-tion. I can only say that I agree with him, and congratulate him for pointing out yet a further form of sejunction, which differs both from my formulation and from Wernicke's original concept.

Erwin Stransky (1877–1962)

Erwin Stransky was born and worked in Vienna, studied neurology and psychiatry in the early years of the century and was awarded a personal chair in psychiatry during the First World War. In 1938 he was stripped of his position because he was Jewish, but was reinstated in 1945.

He was a prolific writer on neurology, mainstream psychiatry and psychotherapy. The article selected for translation here illustrates his attempt to explain schizophrenia both in psychological terms and in the light of what was known at that time of higher cortical disorders. His notion of an 'intrapsychic ataxia' – a dissociation between the intellectual and the emotional functions of the brain – is of particular interest in view of the recent suggestions that hemisphere imbalance might be involved in schizophrenia.

Towards an understanding of certain symptoms of dementia praecox

E. Stransky (1904)

(Zur Auffassung gewisser Symptome der Dementia praecox. *Neurologisches Centralblatt* **23**, 1137–43)

I would like to begin by commenting briefly on a vagrant, charged with attempted theft, who was thought to be simulating mental illness. In support of this view there was a marked contradiction in his behaviour which alternated between a considerable ability to grasp relatively complicated matters and a refusal to respond to the simplest demands. Another factor was the strange contrariness of his spontaneous behaviour.

I could not, at first, make up my mind whether he was simulating or not. There were other factors that argued against it. As Reimann said: 'The decision to simulate mental disorder always requires a driving motive which must be stronger than the fear of those measures which a mental illness brings in its train.' In the present case, no such motive could be detected. According to the information supplied not only by his relatives but also by a fellow-countryman of the patient, an entirely trustworthy informant who knew the family and held an official position in Vienna, there were no grounds for suspecting criminal motives. Neither before nor after his discharge had the patient been in conflict with the law, and since his discharge he has lived quietly with his parents. The minor and somewhat clumsy attempt at theft was off-hand; indeed, nothing about it suggests that it was a planned criminal act. Such thefts are not uncommon in certain forms of mental illness, particularly among patients with general paralysis or hebephrenia who make up such a large proportion of ordinary vagrants.

I rejected the possibility that he might be simulating mental illness in order to escape military service because he was a reservist, who had already completed his military service, and was liable to attend only a few short periods of weapon practice. Even supposing that he wanted to get out of this practice, there is evidence which argues against this. According to his own account, his first symptoms appeared during a sea crossing to America, and he had to be sent straight back to Europe by the fellow-countrymen with whom he had travelled. Such behaviour is highly improbable in one who is seeking to evade military service. Moreover we had independent confirmation that he and his companions were going to America in order to earn more money, and we learned that after his return, when he was called up for his statutory training in weaponry, he did not seek to avoid this duty.

We still have to ask the question whether this could be a case not so much of simulation of a mental illness as of simulation within the framework of a mental illness. The only diagnoses we have to consider in this context are certain hysterical states, in particular Ganser's syndrome. Jung has recently emphasised the important role of strong emotion in the aetiology of these and similar states. In the present case, however, such an assumption is unlikely to apply. It is not that there are no hysterical stigmata. The entire behaviour of the patient and the further course of the illness have little in common with a Ganser syndrome: the nature of his speech disorder is different, there is no emotional factor whatsoever, there are no circumscribed memory defects, and no dim memory of the initial phase of the illness.

For these reasons the differential diagnosis lies between an acute psychosis and the catatonic form of dementia praecox. The former seems to me to be less likely, for the patient presents neither the picture of simple confusion with its prevailing bewilderment, nor that of dream-like hallucinatory confusion such as is found in cases of fully developed amentia. [Amentia was a term used for what we would call acute schizophreniform psychosis, cycloid psychosis, psychogenic psychosis or atypical psychosis, Tr.] It was the striking lack of consistency in the clinical picture that made me suspect a catatonic disorder and not amentia or simulation. His writings also bore the characteristic signs of catatonia: verbigeration, mishmash of words and syllables, perseveration in content and peculiar manneristic flourishes.

Then there was his strange reaction to painful stimuli, to electric stimulation or to simulated threats of such stimulation. Although these procedures, repeated several times, were clearly very painful to him, they produced no change in his psychomotor behaviour, which also argues against simulation. His affective behaviour was suggestive of catatonia. Although apathy was sometimes conspicuous, we cannot exactly say that he was lacking in affect, but what affect he did show was hardly ever consistent with what was going on in his mind. He could not account adequately for his cheerful mien. He would say, for instance, that he did not know where he was and that he felt very strange, but recount all this with a contented laugh. For comparison, we need only think of the anxiety which accompanies amentia, when the patients with this condition no longer grasp their surroundings or do not know at all where they are. In our patient, the motor gestures did not betray the bewilderment that one would expect to correspond with his intellectual state.

We could say that his *noo-psychic state* [Stransky's term for cognitive functions, Tr.] had no *thymo-psychic correlate* [emotional functions, Tr.]. Further, when the florid psychosis abated, the patient showed an unmistakable degree of noo- and thymo-psychic debility. He lacked all initiative and even seemed mentally deficient. I learnt subsequently that this state has persisted. In view of all this evidence I believe I am justified in saying that this is a case of remission occurring in a patient with dementia praecox (catatonic sub-type).

I should now like to turn to those disturbances of conduct and behaviour which resemble in some respects the conditions of asymbolia and apraxia seen in organic brain damage. What springs to mind here is not so much the bewilderment or retardation, which we are accustomed to see in quite different forms of psychosis, but something peculiarly inappropriate, perverse or senseless which interrupts the execution of commonplace acts and might consist of perseveration, inhibition or behaviour such as singing, biting or belching. At the same time some other complicated action, such as counting, can be logically and correctly carried out, either in its entirety or in fragments. This pattern of behaviour, I believe, is typical of that loss of inner consistency which I would venture to call *intrapsychic inco-ordination* or *intrapsychic ataxia*.

I should like to emphasise here that this form of mental disturbance is not the same as that which Wernicke called sejunction (see page 36).

I have two reasons for stressing this point. First, Gross (see page 36), when he wrote about disturbances of coordination in dementia praecox, was merely developing Wernicke's hypothesis of a disturbance in consciousness, which is not what I mean here. Secondly, Wernicke himself, in describing sejunction of consciousness, was referring to a different type of psychological dysfunction. There is a certain parallel between Wernicke's explanation for the inappropriate movements which one sees in many mentally ill patients and my account of the behaviour of patients with dementia praecox. But this is only an analogy, for my starting point was the dissociation of the functional connection between noo- and thymo-psyche in these patients and I emphasised that it is not a question of complete severance of the connection between the two but only of difficulty, uncertainty and inadequacy in their interplay, for which reason I made the comparison with inco-ordination and ataxia.

The central point of my argument turns on a dissociation of the functional connection between noo- and thymo-psyche in such patients. I believe that this dissociation may explain those disorders where there is a discrepancy between affect and mental state. I also believe that one of the characteristic and peculiar aspects of our patient's inaptitude can be put down to a disturbance of attention – not in the generally accepted sense of a straightforward decline in apperception, but a continual, irregular lability of attention governed by the underlying intrapsychic disturbance of coordination. This would account for the capriciousness often found in such patients and their distractibility.

The case I have just described shows just this kind of continual wavering of attention governed by the lack of coordination between the two psychological spheres that leads in the end to emotional and intellectual debility. It is not unusual for patients with dementia praecox to look bewildered, though the dominant affect here was one of imperturbable euphoria that was quite inappropriate to the situation. This was particularly evident when the patient was faced with painful stimuli or simulated threats. Occasionally, one sees the opposite reaction to painful stimuli or threats of attack: the patient will respond with a great expenditure of energy but to so little purpose that he does not succeed in becoming master of the situation. These are the sort of patients who are capable of highly dangerous aggressive acts. One of my patients, when pricked with a needle, would give a terrible scream, writhe in pain and clutch at the examiner's arm, but would in fact take no real defensive action; in the next minute she would strike his hand away sharply and sometimes give him a good pinch. In her rage she would sometimes smilingly destroy folding doors or demolish whole windows. Another patient of mine would suddenly walk slowly and with no particular sign of anger from the end of the garden to the wall of the house, where she would break a pane of glass; on another occasion she would box the doctor's ears for some trifling reason, or smash a glass door because she was supposed to have her hair combed. Yet shortly after such a fit of rage she would allow a painful stimulus to be applied without showing any reaction at all. It seems to me that my hypothesis of inco-ordination explains such traits much better than any assumption of absolute dissociation or sejunction, as put forward by Wernicke. The core of the disturbance seems to me to be the ataxic instability in thymo- and noo-psychic relationships. One should also note that the confused speech of these patients, like the rest of their psychomotor behaviour, bears characteristic signs of inco-ordination in the above sense.

I hope the foregoing remarks may have helped to explain the difference between my views on the psychological basis of dementia praecox and those of Gross and Wernicke. The present case, with its many interesting features, has given me the opportunity of pointing out these differences. What is of most practical interest in the case is the characteristic symptomatology, which shows how easy it is, in the absence of a careful analysis, to diagnose catatonic states as simulation, which has many forensic implications. I would also point out as noteworthy the extensive remission which occurred in this case.

Wilhelm Weygandt (1870–1939)

Wilhelm Weygandt was born in Wiesbaden and first studied psychology under Wundt in Leipzig before taking up medicine and eventually psychiatry. He worked with Kraepelin in Heidelberg and was appointed a professor first in Wurzburg and then Hamburg. He was particularly interested in child psychiatry and mental retardation, and the following extract sets out his ideas on certain similarities between schizophrenia and mental retardation. It also contains a searching critique of Freud's ideas on psychosis.

Critical comments on the psychology of dementia praecox

W. Weygandt (1907)

(Kritische Bemerkungen zur Psychologie der Dementia praecox. *Monatsschrift für Psychiatrie und Neurologie* **22**, 289–301)

Freud's theories have become a kind of fashion. His views have been praised and glorified as if he were a second Galileo. Surprisingly enough, Breuer is seldom mentioned, although in 1896 Freud credited him with the main achievement when he spoke of his significant discovery of the factors that determine the symptoms of hysteria.

Critical discussion can be no more than a warning to the uninitiated, since the adherents and builders of this theory have immured themselves against criticism behind a virtually impregnable wall, so that any attempt to refute their argument may well seem useless before it is started. For this is how it goes: only if you yourself have made frequent use of the psychoanalytical method and, like Freud, have carried out prolonged and patient observation of daily life, hysteria and dreams from your own personal point of view – only then may you venture to attempt a refutation. With such reservations anyone can of course proclaim the most fantastic theories. If an investigator uses a defective staining method, which alters and damages the nerve cell substances or its nucleus and then publishes new findings that apply to every kind of cerebral disorder, must one really first make thorough tests of the defective method on all similar cerebral disorders before one may utter a critical word on the significance of such findings?

I have certainly not carried out prolonged and patient observation of many patients who are hysterical in Freud's sense of the term in the manner that the above passage would imply. Nor have Freud and his followers conducted long and patient observation of cases of dementia praecox: their publications on this disorder were based in many instances on one or just a few patients. We do, however, share an interest in the psychology of the dream, which I have long been interested in, and as Freud, in his great work *The Interpretation of Dreams*, saw the dream as the most important of all abnormal psychological happenings, it is worth looking first at this particular field. This is especially relevant to the psychoanalytic notion of dementia praecox because as early as 1893 Freud was claiming that 'hallucinatory madness' was a 'flight into psychosis', an attempt to find in the dream-like delirium of illness what was lacking to a person in real life.

Criticism must begin with Freud's main formulation that 'the dream is a wish-fulfilment'. First of all, it is rather arbitrary to see the dream as an entity at all, since one is always dealing with only a part of the totality of dream images, a part that has been torn from a larger context which has disappeared from memory. The term 'wish fulfilment' would perhaps do credit to the psychology of a novelist, but in a scientific analysis must itself be subjected to a more penetrating examination and brought more into line with elementary psychological phenomena.

In my view, when consciousness is lowered, the first consequence is a cessation of the purposive ideas of waking thought and the intrusion into dream consciousness of other factors which were excluded from the conscious mind. In the forefront of these factors are all kinds of sensory stimuli, in particular those of the sensory organs. Next come ideas which have been repressed for some time and which now return to consciousness, their return being governed by mood. Mood is of paramount importance, and according to the prevailing mood we get pleasant or unpleasant ideas. However, such pleasant and unpleasant feelings are accompanied by an effort to surmount them. Since the impulse to surmount an unpleasantly coloured situation is not usually translated into the motor sphere, we are left only with the idea of the situation that has been successfully overcome – which corresponds to Freud's wish-fulfilment. But the cause of the unpleasantness usually continues during sleep, so that often the idea of fulfilment is succeeded immediately by one of lack or disappointment. Relevant examples are dreams of thirst and dreams of bladder discomfort: in both we find the image of overcoming the unpleasant situation, by drinking or urinating, but this often gives way to disillusionment in that we are still thirsty or want to pass water, only to be followed by a further image of wish fulfilment which may appear for a second or even third time, leading to the well-known phenomenon of repetitive dreams.

Viewed in this way the wish fulfilment of dreams becomes to some extent plausible, but it is still incorrect to see in it anything at all basic to the true nature of dreams. Often enough, unpleasantly coloured ideas are not overcome in dreams. Abraham, one of Freud's main disciples, moreover, was not being very precise when he spoke of a female patient with hallucinations who heard a voice telling her that she would live long, have children, marry and receive an inheritance; he called this wish fulfilment, but in fact it concerned only images of the future, not an image of fulfilled expectations.

Freud regards infancy and sexuality as particularly fertile sources of dream images. I certainly concede the latter point. Fourteen years ago I pointed out that it was in fact sexual sensations which first directed my attention to the relationship between sensory stimuli and dream images. Their influence, however, is not preponderant, though individual differences in regard to sexuality are of course enormous. I am strongly of the opinion that it is sexual sensations that are principally involved in dreams, not just sexual memories.

While commending Freud's endeavour to uncover the roots of every element in every group of dream images, I think he goes far too far in his search for meaning, as when he traces the dream of flying to the rocking of childhood, whereas it would be much more relevant to trace it back to the sensations of breathing and of balance. The fanciful dream interpreter, Scherner, whom Freud criticised, was in fact on the right track when he associated the dream of flying with the sensation of breathing freely, though he was also naive enough to mention the connection between the wings (*Flügel*) in the dream and the two lobes or 'wings' (*Flügel*) of the lungs.

One dream which typifies Freud's speculative interpretation is the dream of a lady who saw three lions in the desert (one of them laughing), of whom she was not afraid. Freud analysed the dream in the following tortuous way. The neutral cause of the dream was a sentence in an English exercise that ran: 'the mane is the adornment of the lion'. The lady's father had a beard that somewhat resembled a mane. Her English teacher was called Miss Lyons (lions = *Löwen*) and a friend had sent her a copy of Löwe's ballads. 'These are the three lions – why should she be afraid of them?' When we look at the contrived way in which the three lions are interpreted, we might well think ourselves transplanted into the world of popular dream interpretation;

the dream itself – we need only think of the Biblical example of dreams of seven fat and seven lean cows – is in the juxtaposition of its many component ideas almost as free and variable as, say, delirium tremens with its confusion of delusional perceptions.

This excessive search for connections permeates the most diverse studies of Freud and his followers and makes them almost unreadable to those who seek assured relationships and not just frivolous echoes of the images in question. Still in the genre of the dream of the three lions, we have the case of the hysterical girl whose lover once tried to possess her and who subsequently developed a stiff hysterical paralysis of the arm, based on the impression of the stiff, hard penis. The aim of all scientific endeavour, namely to advance to certainty, leaving faith and the acceptance of mere probabilities behind, is here abandoned in favour of chasing after vague, frivolous connections which in their tortuous construction are of no more value than the attempted interpretations and explanations that take place in forecasting the results of a Papal election.

Freud's attempts to understand hysteria are similarly flawed. There is, as in his dream interpretations, an excessive concern with the sexual sphere. Nor must one forget the factor of memory falsification, which plays a much greater part than is usually assumed. Other sources of error are the in-depth examination and the asking of leading questions, however much investigators in the Freudian tradition may guard against them. Freud's doctrine is both reprehensible because of its arbitrariness of interpretation and commendable because of its emphasis on encouraging the patient to talk things out: for these two reasons one has to agree with Hoche when he said, in the words of Lessing, 'what is new in it is not good and what is good is not new'. In fact the psychological side of our work as specialists in nervous and mental disorders is and always has been much more securely based on an understanding examination of the patient's range of ideas, and on helping and accompanying him in his recollections, than on suggestion and hypnosis.

It may be admitted that unpleasant subconscious memory fragments do play a part in hysterical mood disturbances, and that the unpleasantness can most quickly be overcome by exposing it and talking freely about it. But far greater scepticism is called for when the same method is applied to the mental processes of dementia praecox.

Freud tried to do this as early as 1896, asserting that dementia paranoides (schizophrenia) was a defence neuro-psychosis which, like hysteria and obsessional states, arose from repression of painful

memories, and that the form of the patients' symptoms was determined by the content of their repressed ideas.

The word 'determined' is of course open to different interpretations.
It can be equated with 'conditioned' or used directly to mean 'caused'.
It should be emphasised here that Freud's successors, who in their
analysis of hysteria admit that there is just possibly an element of
predisposition present, also distinguish between 'determined' and
'caused' and concede that another, perhaps toxic, factor may possibly
play a part.

Freud, of course, thought of a deeper relationship, as we can see
from one case that he described. A thirty-year-old woman became
mentally ill and thought that she was being observed especially while
undressing. She experienced sensations in her abdomen which she
regarded as being caused by indecent thoughts on the part of the
parlourmaid. She had visual hallucinations of male and female genitals
and thought that her own genitals were being observed.

Though Freud stresses that the hallucinations began when the
patient saw other female patients naked in the communal bathroom,
he admits that she was then already ill. She now reported that as a child
of six she had taken all her clothes off in front of her little brother,
without feeling ashamed, but that between the ages of eight and
seventeen she had been ashamed of her nakedness in the bath, in front
of her mother, her sister and the doctor. The onset of her morbid mood
disturbance is now said to have coincided with a quarrel with her
husband and her brother. The idea that people wished her ill came to
her because of something said by a visiting sister-in-law.

I see nothing to dispute in this: a female patient with a developing
mood disorder and sensory delusions formed a connection between
sexual sensations and the disturbing experience of seeing several
naked women in the bathroom, whereupon she had visual hallucinations of genitalia. I can accept that in response to questioning she
thought she remembered childhood experiences of taking all her
clothes off. What in my view cannot be reliably asserted, however, is
that these images would have returned into her consciousness without
the doctor's probing questions, or that they played any particular part
in influencing her morbid ideas.

Among Freud's followers it was Jung in particular who took up this
concept of dementia praecox, which he has tried to develop further in
his interesting book. He too, however, concedes that the illness may
have an underlying physical cause that goes far beyond anything
psychological.

After presenting the numerous attempts that have been made to unite the phenomena of dementia praecox in one formulation, be it as a breakdown of association or consciousness or personality, or as a form of abnormal fixation with apathy and apperceptive deficiency, Jung emphasises one fact which Freud and Gross had already noted, namely that dissociated trains of ideas do play a part. Quoting numerous examples he tries to show that every affectively coloured happening becomes a 'complex', an affectively coloured group of conscious processes which tend to harden into a single entity.

While the kernel of hysteria thus consists in a complex which is never quite overcome, so that one may assume a causal relationship between complex and illness (a suitable predisposition also being assumed), Jung takes a different view of dementia praecox. In this disorder one or several complexes have become permanently fixated. It is not clear whether the complex causes or triggers the illness in a predisposed subject, or whether it only determines symptoms at the moment of onset of the illness. In cases in which a strong affect exists at the start of the illness one is tempted to attach causal significance to the complex. There is one proviso, however, in that the complex may generate a factor X (? a toxin) which contributes to the disturbance. A further reservation concedes the possibility that X might also be of primary origin. From the standpoint of physiological psychology, both parallelism and the theory of reciprocal action, there would seem to be something wrong here, in that this problematical toxin is viewed as a highly developed body which attaches itself throughout to psychic processes, particularly to those which are affectively coloured.

The way is now open to develop an explanation covering the wide variety of symptoms found in dementia praecox – the so-called train of thought, the blockage and suppression, the negativism and stereotypy.

Why is it then that we struggle so hard against accepting this doctrine that has been expounded by reputable authors? Are there parts of the theory which may still be upheld and explained in a way that contradicts less glaringly the concept of dementia praecox which hitherto prevailed?

The findings revealed by neuroanatomical studies, genetic surveys and the investigation of endogenous factors have led psychiatrists to regard psychological factors, except in the case of hysteria, as able to colour an illness but not determine its essential nature. Dementia praecox, in particular, is more and more regarded as an illness based on some metabolic disturbance. Frequent analogies are made with general paralysis of the insane. So any attempt to view dementia praecox as a psychological disorder in its essential cause, a defence neuro-psychosis determined by the repression of painful complexes, can be reduced to absurdity by following it to its logical conclusion. It is like attributing general paralysis of the insane to a psychosexual trauma in adolescence or senile dementia perhaps to masturbation. Jung was well aware of this danger. One way which he dealt with it was to introduce the factor X. He also pointed out, rightly, that clinicians have known for a long time that psychogenic symptoms can occur in organic disturbances. He did, however, claim that somehow psychological distress could induce organic changes in the brain – that factor X could be itself produced by purely psychological processes. That I dispute.

If the psychoanalytic view that psychological disturbance can be primary is unacceptable, is there scope for admitting that the content of a psychosis is largely made up of images from long forgotten days? I myself do not think that this is true of dreams, hysteria or of dementia praecox. The emergence of everyday material is, in my view, more likely in all mental disorders. We need think only of the occupational delirium of the alcoholic. The source of delusional perceptions lies often enough in images that are borrowed from the immediate present. And I recall a patient, with an illness of recent onset, who a few weeks after Röntgen's first publication on X-rays sought to account for his hallucinations on the basis of such concepts, which certainly did not emanate from his childhood. In general paralysis, and to an even greater extent in senile dementia, patients usually do hark back to their early days, frequently to their first years at school, and the same often happens in dreams. It is also true in many cases of hysteria and dementia praecox. We must, however, dispute the generalisation of this assumption, the artificial interpretations given of particular circumstances, and above all the attempt to attach to such factors a determinative or aetiological significance.

In conclusion I should like to put forward a tentative explanation of dementia praecox of my own which might cover the resurgence of memories, the infantile traits and the marked motor phenomena. I would suggest that so far as the organic side is concerned the most plausible concept is one of autotoxic damage affecting genetically predisposed brains.

In an earlier paper, based on a study of old cases of dementia praecox whose acute state had occurred almost fifty years earlier, I stressed an often-quoted finding which was particularly clearcut in my group, namely that while intellectual assets may be well preserved the capacity to utilise them is lost; will and affect in particular are dulled and the best and most personal of human attributes, initiative and self-esteem, disappear. Using Wundt's terminology, I spoke then of 'apperceptive dementia'.

By studying patients with mental deficiency and phenomena which occur at certain stages of normal child development I was then struck by a similarity between the pattern of movement of such children and the movement disorder that is seen in dementia praecox. Rhythmic movements and grimacing, for example, occurred in all three groups. Echo symptoms, and more rarely command automatisms, were also seen. Even speech disorder, particularly vergiberation and neologisms, could occur. Normal speech development in the child passes through three stages which may be described briefly as crying, babbling and speaking, or in other words the phase of unco-ordinated discharge of motor impulses using the musculature of speech, then the phase of oral sounds which the child begins to apprehend and modify without any inner understanding, and finally conceptual speech. I would suggest that so far as the mental development of retarded idiots is concerned, in cases of hydrocephaly or microcephaly for example, speech development stops essentially at the stage of babbling, or even at the lowest stage of all, crying; it is much the same with other motor expressions though these can of course undergo still more specific modifications.

So far as dementia praecox is concerned I would suggest that the toxic influence first damages at its deepest level that most personal quality which must operate if the psychic functioning of the individual is to remain intact. As the disturbance grows more severe, the patient regresses to a lower developmental level and his motor and oral behaviour approach those phases of child development, or those states in idiocy determined by an inhibition of cerebral development.

To this extent I would agree with Jungian concepts, according to which when personality is disturbed, when there is apperceptive dementia, suppressed images, forgotten memories and old, dead emotions penetrate again into consciousness, replacing the purposive ideas governed by the personality. If the illness spreads, and there is a further loss of active attention and will, the more severe motor symptoms come to the fore, this process corresponding to the normal developmental phase in which motor impulses are dominant and not controlled by ideas – the phase of babbling and rhythmic movement.

I shall be reproached for simply replacing one hypothesis by another. Yet science cannot proceed without hypotheses. The question is only how far we may rely upon them. According to Wundt, a hypothesis should present an assumption about the true nature and relationship of certain intuitively perceived facts. Critical examination will judge my attempt to take facts derived from clinical observation of patients and from the observation of children and to juxtapose these facts in the form of particular symptoms. The Freudian theory of dementia praecox, on the other hand, starts with the uncontrollable expressions of irresponsible patients and goes on to make general statements about long-vanished, affectively-coloured complexes which have ostensibly been recalled into consciousness; such complexes are then said to be of possible causal significance in the whole dementing process and to play a particularly important part in the development of motor symptoms which in fact are encountered just as frequently in born imbeciles. Surely this argument is a dubious one, which is not in keeping with the total content of our experience.

Joseph Berze (1866–1958)

Joseph Berze was born in Vienna where he spent all his professional life. His clinical posts were in forensic psychiatry but he was a prolific writer on the causes, psychology and treatment of all aspects of psychosis.

The article selected here contains his views on the nature of schizophrenia. It represents a view of mental illness which was at odds with the ideas of Kraepelin and Bleuler, and is notable for the emphasis placed on general cognitive impairment, particularly the defect of attention.

Primary insufficiency of mental activity
J. Berze (1914)
(Chapter 4 of *Die Primäre Insuffizienz der Psychischen Aktivität*. Leipzig: F. Deuticke)

Many patients with a mental illness report that they have noticed a decline or weakness in consciousness. When we try to understand what is meant by such statements, however, we are not helped much by the usual definitions of consciousness which generally refer to it as the 'knowledge of a process going on within us' or as the 'act of experiencing psychic phenomena'. Such definitions are incorrect because consciousness can differ in intensity, whereas a 'knowledge of a process' or an 'act' either exists or does not exist.

The possibility of differences in intensity means that consciousness must be a process itself. Further evidence for this lies in the fact that the words we use to describe the phenomena of consciousness – 'becoming conscious of', 'making conscious' – point to the working of a process and not just 'all-or-nothing' knowledge of something. Consciousness is best regarded, in my view, in terms of the operation of certain forces which underlies purposeful mental activity.

Insufficient mental activity causes a reduction in the level of consciousness (purposeful mental activity) as well as a reduction in spontaneous activity and reactivity. A mild reduction in spontaneous activity will manifest itself as a diminished capacity for thinking efficiently. So far as reactivity is concerned, the decline does not become obvious until the defect is fairly severe, since, in general, reactions call for a much lower level of functional preparedness.

General effects of insufficient activity

In mild degress of insufficiency the chief effect will be a diminution of spontaneous and purposeful activity. Patients suffering from this degree of insufficient activity will notice that the general clarity of consciousness, their will, their awareness of themselves, their attention, their capacity to think clearly, their perceptual powers, their comprehension and their memory are all impaired. It also accounts for many of their delusional ideas. Because reactivity is hardly affected with this level of insufficient mental activity, patients are aware only that their reactions appear more strained, although they are not reduced in intensity. This may be experienced as feelings of passivity, discomfort, unpleasantness or suffering.

If the insufficiency is more severe, it can produce a paradoxical enhancement of reactions because reactivity is affected less than purposeful and spontaneous activity. The stimulation of memories by casual events in the environment may dominate the mind whereas more energetic mental activity may be in abeyance. They may report passive, involuntary thinking – thoughts or thought processes which come into being without their volition or even against their will. They compare themselves to automatons or instruments. Memories may take complete precedence over perceptions. A feeling of suffering usually accompanies these experiences.

If the insufficiency progresses still further, a condition may arise in which the individual is no longer able to cope with sensory stimuli at all. They appear so powerful by comparison with ideas generated from within that there ensues a complete loss of the sense of self. The patient has become an automaton: perception and memory have become so hopelessly intermingled that he is wholly confused in his conduct and expression. This accounts for the acute, florid stage of a psychosis.

Eventually the insufficiency may be so severe that even reactivity is reduced to a minimum. Although reactivity makes much less demand on functional preparedness in the intentional sphere, it nevertheless still presupposes a certain minimal level of consciousness.

Varieties of disturbed consciousness

Psychiatrists who have not understood that consciousness can vary in degree believe that there is only one type of disturbance. They speak of clouding of consciousness or clouding of the sensorium. Even Bleuler favoured this concept. His passage on the subject of consciousness, which takes up barely half a page in his otherwise wide-ranging work (Bleuler, 1911), begins with the words: 'The term disturbance of consciousness, which to a certain extent is the equivalent of the old term clouding of consciousness, corresponds to no clear concept'. His further remarks show that for him the two terms are not just 'to a certain extent equivalent' but completely identical.

Many patients with dementia praecox, however, recognise that their consciousness can be disturbed without being clouded, and that this takes the form of a reduction of psychic activity – a purely quantitative defect. Genuine clouding of consciousness *can* occur in dementia praecox when the insufficient activity is particularly severe. Clouding of consciousness can also occur in other conditions and for other reasons. In toxic confusional states and genuine organic dementia a pathological overstimulation of the sensory regions of the brain may occur giving rise to a breakdown in consciousness. We can therefore distinguish at least two varieties of clouding of consciousness or confusional state: one where the intrinsic level of mental activity is too weak to accommodate sensory input – as in dementia praecox – the other where the sensory input is itself pathologically enhanced due to pathological irritation – as in toxic confusional states.

Depersonalisation

We attribute the insufficiency of activity and the ensuing weakness of consciousness to an underlying impoverishment of an individual's beliefs and drives. Since the self is a product of a collection of these motives and drives then any deficiency in this sphere must affect the sense of self as well as that of the outside world. Why some patients experience this as a weakness of consciousness and others more as a change in the sense of self is unclear, though it must be added that patients do not as a rule draw a sharp distinction between the two concepts. The disturbances of self awareness may be of different degrees of severity, up to complete depersonalisation. Patients can discern the most varied aspects of this defect and attach great importance to it. And despite his claim that there is only one type of disturbance of consciousness, Bleuler recognises in his clinical experience the frequency and varied nature of this phenomenon in his patients with dementia praecox. He quotes the case of a woman, for example, who had to make an effort to 'find my own self for a few short moments'; others 'had lost their individual self' . . .

Personality change

The precise clinical picture of personality change depends on whether the defect in activity is constant or variable. Bleuler believed that complete changes of personality were usually associated with severe grades of dementia. In my view, however, many such cases show no dementia at all. If the defect in activity is intermittent, then the personality change will also fluctuate. I have in my care a patient whom I have been able to observe for years. He is in fact a captain in the army, aged 50, who goes through phases in which he believes that he is a 25–year–old pregnant woman, just about to give birth. Another patient of mine, who also suffers intermittent insufficiency of activity, alternates between relative normality and a hallucinatory state. When he is in the 'normal' phase he realises that what he experienced and did in the 'hallucinatory' phase was 'pure rubbish'. His 'normal self' regards his 'hallucinatory self' as a 'slave' 'playing a passive role' and as having given himself up to 'alien thoughts'. While actually in the 'hallucinatory state' he does not know that he is acting like a slave. It is only later, when his consciousness is again 'normal', that he understandably concludes that, since in the 'hallucinatory state' he had to act in a way that was contrary to his real intentions, he was being robbed of his freedom of thought, action and deliberation. In the 'hallucinatory state' one can say that he has already undergone a change of personality, though this new personality is not yet quite consolidated. Eventually it may be even given a name, as in another case of mine, who called it 'Prince L, grandson of the Kaiser' . . .

As personality is the end result of a complex interaction of drives and beliefs, held together by the action of the will, then if the general level of mental activity diminishes and the will weakens this collection of different complexes of drives and beliefs may fragment. Pseudo-personalities, such as the 'hallucinatory self' and 'Prince L', mentioned above, may become permanent. Further personalities may appear, as the fragmented complexes become more independent, and a patient may continually wander from one to another. Sometimes external stimuli may act as the trigger because, as I mentioned earlier, a decrease in overall mental activity can lead to external stimuli having undue influence. One of my patients, for example, while leafing through an old magazine, passed through a succession of extraordinarily different personalities, each founded on the illustrations and images encountered in the magazine.

Split personality

The interruption of ego continuity by pseudo-personalities, such as we saw in our discussion of personality change, should not be confused with the phenomenon known as 'splitting' of the personality.

Wernicke called this symptom the 'breakdown of individuality . . . The higher associations are no longer all combined in one unified ego . . . The patient consists simultaneously of a number of different personalities'. He considered that the basic defect, which he called sejunction, consisted of 'a break in continuity, a structural loosening of associations, which must correspond to the loss of certain associative performance'.

The term 'split personality' is more often used nowadays, and has replaced Wernicke's term 'breakdown of individuality'. It is usually understood to mean the simultaneous existence of two or more personalities. These personalities represent elements split off from the real personality.

Bleuler's concept of 'splitting' is quite different and has little to do with simultaneous awareness of sub-personalities. This can be explained by the fact that he tended to underestimate the significance of the role of consciousness in mental life. For Bleuler it was quite incidental whether a complex was at any given moment consciously known or not. The only important point about 'splitting', in his formulation, was the simultaneous existence of at least one *unconscious* complex competing with one *conscious* complex.

For our part we would adhere firmly to the original meaning of the concept and we therefore believe that one should speak of 'splitting' only when there is evidence that two or more personalities are existing simultaneously in consciousness. It must be added, however, that even if the occurrence of splitting in this sense can scarcely be doubted – Kraepelin, Jaspers and others have described clear-cut cases – the phenomenon is not common. In many instances the 'splitting' is illusory – a misperception of what is in fact a rapidly developing change of personality. Many cases that have been reported in the literature come under this heading. They should be regarded as a dialogue between several personalities. In such instances, the patient experiences himself as being forcibly given the delusional idea of being split, of a splitting of his personality.

The following case illustrates the typical way in which a split personality is usually manifest.

A female factory hand, single, aged 47, was admitted for the first time in February 1913. She had suffered for many years from a delusion of persecution and for ten years had been fit only for light household duties. From time to time she would appear quite normal but then suddenly and with no apparent cause delusional ideas of persecution accompanied by anxiety would appear.

On admission she was correctly orientated in place and time, had average intelligence and there was no memory disturbance. She complained of 'talk going on in her head', and sometimes she would hear strange voices, some of which she could make out clearly, and one of which was her doctor, Dr K. She blamed her experiences on a powder which her mother had given her years earlier. She did not know why her mother had given her this powder, and was not sure whether it was to do her good or harm. She said that she was 'not clever enough to be able to decide which'. She could not think like other people, believing that from her early days she had not been as good as others at thinking.

On one occasion when the talking was going on in her head she said she was 'outside herself' and did not know what she was saying. The talking was not usually loud but she always heard it clearly and 'directly in her head'. Sometimes the talking reached such a pitch that she fell asleep. Its content was partly nonsensical, partly threatening. Often the things that were said were quite new and quite unknown to her. She would be told that she would be executed or hanged, and had a 'feeling' as if an axe were swinging over her head. When her eyes were shut she had a white light in her head, and when the talking was going on she had a dull feeling in her head. She also thought that the talking in her head seemed to be talking to itself.

At times she would say, 'I am an officer of the Guard of Honour in the Hofburg Palaces. My three brothers are inside me. We men are able to say things that she won't admit.' She went on speaking of herself in the third person. She would dance around clumsily, saying that she felt an urge to sing or dance.

She left the institution shortly afterwards but was admitted again in November 1913. According to informants she had recently been cheerful and lively, skipping around and dressing up like a flirtatious young girl. She had made senseless purchases in order to satisfy passing whims, considered herself 'smart', wanted to be admired by everyone and wanted 'a lovely house in a sunny situation'. She spoke disrespectfully about her relatives and composed rhymes.

On admission she was oriented in time and place and remembered clearly her previous stay in the institution. She was distractible, restless and talkative, and had a compulsion to speak in rhymes: 'One, two and here I stand . . . here is she and me . . . me too, I've come to you'. Sometimes she was very restless, protesting sharply about what she regarded as unnatural treatment. She was coquettish and affected, and spoke at times in correct German but then lapsed into the local dialect, with coarse expressions.

She announced that there was an assortment of different people inside her – an officer of the Guard of Honour, Ernst Ritter von Pöheim, Dr K., a conference of doctors and a men's choral society. She later said that she had come to the institution because Lt von Pöheim, an officer of the Guard of Honour in Baden, was within her in an 'electric assortment'. When answering questions she would lose the thread of what she was saying and resort to neologisms, speaking in rhyme with no regard for the meaning of what she was saying. When asked if she herself were present in these assortments she explained: 'I am as I am, I am not present in any assortment.' On the other hand she would talk about herself in the third person, referring to herself as 'the girl', identifying herself with the 'girl' and saying that 'the girl' often has a conversation with Lt von Pöheim: 'The girl is not there when the assortments are there. The officer is like a shadow beside her when the girl is there. The girl is always trying to think. But when the officer is there the girl only exists for those around her. The assortments used to be there only rarely, now they are always there. I feel I haven't got the strength any more to oppose the will of other people.'

When asked how she knew that Dr K. was speaking inside her, she replied, 'I feel it; he always begins like that; I attract his will; if you come under another person's will, then you feel nothing but that will. He's doing all sorts of silly things. I can't help it, I have to laugh. He is in me, very strongly. There is always an officer beside me, two of them, Dr K. and the officer, are talking to one another. He says, Ernst, she is a dear girl. He lies beside me in bed, in full uniform, without a sword. He is lying in his clothes like a shadow beside me. I am sometimes my own will. Then he comes up to me quickly and passes through my will. Sometimes he lets me go but when he is there I cannot free myself. As I am quite under his will, the will changes, the two wills cannot work together. Sometimes they are side by side, but there is only one will. Herr P. has just said I have sacrificed the bread.'

This patient evidently distinguished between her total personality – her true self ('I am as I am') – and the part-personalities – the 'assortments'. These assortments do not in general have the character of a dominant personality but are described as strange personalities – 'in me'. Only one of the assortment is treated by the patient as if she identifies herself, her true self, with it, namely the one whom she describes as 'the girl'. When she feels she is 'the girl', she speaks like a young girl who wants to act elegantly – speaks in correct German, presents herself as proper, coquettish and droll, and flirts with the officer.

We are justified in speaking here of a splitting of personality, a breaking away of the 'assortment' from the dominant personality, since the patient recognises the assortments for what they are at the moment when she experiences them. This means that her own true personality is present at the same time as the assortment, and even when 'the girl' is substituting as the dominant personality it too is apart from and yet simultaneous with the remainder of the assortment.

References

Bleuler, E. (1911) Dementia Praecox oder die Gruppe der Schizophrenien. In *Handbuch der Geisteskrankheiten*, ed. G. Aschaffenburg. Leipzig: F. Deuticke.

Eugen Bleuler (1857–1939)

Eugen Bleuler was born in a Swiss village near Zurich, of farming stock. He studied medicine in Zurich and after a short period in Paris with Charcot and a brief stay in London to study neuropathology he returned to Zurich where he remained for the rest of his life, becoming director of the internationally renowned Burghölzli Clinic.

Bleuler first introduced the term schizophrenia in 1908, in the following article which has never been translated into English before. He suggested that this term was more appropriate than dementia praecox. His monograph on schizophrenia published in 1911 was only translated into English in 1950 and is now out of print. The current extract therefore provides a useful summary of his views on schizophrenia.

The prognosis of dementia praecox: the group of schizophrenias

E. Bleuler (1908)

(Die Prognose der Dementia Praecox – Schizophreniegruppe.
Allgemeine Zeitschrift für Psychiatrie **65**, 436–64)

Introduction

In using the term dementia praecox I would like it to mean what the creator of the concept meant it to mean. To treat the subject from any other point of view would serve no purpose, but I would like to emphasise that Kraepelin's dementia praecox is not necessarily either a form of dementia or a disorder of early onset. For this reason, and because there is no adjective or noun that can be derived from the term dementia praecox, I am taking the liberty of using the word *schizophrenia* to denote Kraepelin's concept. I believe that the tearing apart or splitting of psychic functions is a prominent symptom of the whole group and I will give my reasons for this elsewhere.

With the help of two doctoral students, Wolfsohn and Zablocka, I have taken the records of 647 schizophrenics admitted to Burghölzli over a period of eight years and studied them with particular reference to prognosis . . .

Two points must first be emphasised: not only does prognosis depend on the illness which we diagnose and name according to its symptoms, but it is also determined by a large number of other factors, the effects of which are interwoven and may even cancel each other out. We must therefore make up our minds to consider separately the individual factors and their influences.

The concept of prognosis itself includes many and varied sub-concepts, contained in the following questions:

Will the patient deteriorate intellectually?

What form will this deterioration take (hebephrenic, catatonic, paranoid)?

How far will it progress?

How quickly will it progress?

Will the symptoms remit? Which symptoms? To what extent? How soon?

Will the illness recur, or will there be new and progressively deteriorating attacks?

General and specific prognosis

There is also the question of the difference between a *general* prognosis for the condition as a whole, and a *specific* prognosis for each individual patient. If each sub-group had its own precise, definite prognosis, then there would be no need to consider specific, individual prognoses, because by knowing to which sub-group a patient belonged one would know the patient's precise prognosis. Unfortunately, except for sub-groups such as chronic catatonia, where patients have been chronically ill for years, the general prognosis of a sub-group is as vague as that of the whole illness. It is a general truth that, whatever form the illness may take initially, catatonic symptoms may later supervene, though catatonic disorders, provided they are not acute and transitory, tend to remain catatonic throughout. The same is true of the paranoid sub-group and subjects with delusions of influence. The ideal situation would, of course, be to understand fully the general prognosis of every sub-group.

The general prognosis of dementia praecox is clear to anyone who has grasped Kraepelin's concept. It deals only with qualitative or directional aspects and points towards a specific kind of state to which we give the vague and far too general name of dementia. The general prognosis does not specify how long the disease process takes or how severe the final dementia will be. There is so much individual variation that a 'specific' prognosis is required in virtually every case.

In the present state of our knowledge this specific prognosis amounts virtually to a temporal prognosis, one which would estimate the duration of the illness before the onset of dementia. This quantitative prognosis cannot be too sharply distinguished from the qualitative, directional prognosis, and one has to be content with what Kahlbaum in his day established for catatonia: the process can come to a standstill and equally well resume its progress at any stage of the disease.

The incurability of schizophrenia

If we understand this clearly, then the contentious question of recovery in dementia praecox loses much of its significance. If the dementia comes to an early standstill the patient may seem both to the layman and to many psychiatrists to have recovered. Indeed, many patients can be regarded as cured in the social sense of the term. If no acute attack has occurred, then such cases must remain latent, and latent schizophrenia is quite common, to judge by those patients who are admitted briefly to hospital only on account of random and transient disturbances caused by some unfavourable life event. The large number of schizophrenics who marry after a spell in hospital, and are regarded as healthy, points in the same direction. In my view many of Magnan's 'degenerates' and many paranoid personality disorders described by other authors are misdiagnosed schizophrenics.

It is a matter of individual opinion whether these stationary and improved states, in which the patient is capable of resuming his former life, should be regarded as cures. The decision depends on many factors. One of the most important is the time which the doctor has available for determining the state of the patient on discharge. My own experience leads me at all events to agree with Aschaffenburg's view that in schizophrenia there is no cure in the sense of *restitutio ad integram*. Although the large majority of schizophrenics who have passed through an institution may live permanently outside it and are regarded for the most part as healthy, whenever I have been able to examine any of those who have been pronounced cured I have found a residue of the illness. The diagnosis of a cure has often been rash, in that the discharged patients, without having changed in any way, have speedily had to be readmitted to an institution. Personally I have never treated a patient who has proved on close examination to be entirely free of signs of the illness.

I know patients whose achievements in life have been outstanding, but even these I would not regard as cured. They include business men who independently build up large and successful businesses, civil servants, parsons, a poet and a scholar of international renown. The last of these had suffered two attacks of catatonia before writing a new scientific work. It was a pleasure to discuss scientific matters with him even when he was still suffering from genuine delusional ideas. But when I finally considered him completely ready to resume work, he was still making crude logical mistakes when one spoke to him about the complexes which had played a part in his illness. I would not like to accept as a genuine cure a state in which some parts of the mental apparatus are permanently inaccessible to logic. I can appreciate, however, how physicians who are not used to looking for such phenomena attest many cures.

In the psychological sphere we find that when there is an exacerbation of the illness the ideas from an earlier attack regularly return in some form or other, which also shows that residual mental symptoms of the illness cannot have been completely overcome.

When the disease process flares up, it is more correct, in my view, to talk in terms of deteriorating attacks, rather than its recurrence. Of course the term recurrence is more comforting to a patient and his relatives than the notion of progressively deteriorating attacks.

Time-course of the disease

Although a precise prognosis of the dementing process is impossible at the present time, one may still identify the factors which govern its time-course.

These factors include the important but as yet unknown personal characteristics that can be grouped together under the term disposition. Heredity and the level of mental energy – the only constituents of disposition which are at present recognised – are irrelevant so far as prognosis is concerned.

I have already pointed out that we do not know whether or not the time-course depends upon the sub-group of the illness.

Random external influences must, however, also be relevant and, other things being equal, the patient who from inclination or necessity leads an irregular life which exposes him to many emotional ups and downs is more likely to become ill again than one who lives quietly. In two of my cases a definite recurrence was associated with a chance encounter with a former sweetheart. I have no doubt, too, that treatment counts for a good deal. The sooner the patients can be restored to an ordinary life and the less they are allowed to withdraw into the world of their own ideas, the sooner do they become socially functional. I have not yet observed that deprivations and excesses contribute to a poorer prognosis, but alcohol has an indirect effect, in that it makes it impossible for even mild cases of schizophrenia to function in society.

All these factors must be the subject of detailed investigation, but before committing ourselves to an individual prognosis of the time-course we must first make a precise assessment of the *degree of dementia* or, in other words, of the *aspects of a case which are no longer susceptible to remission*.

The nature of the dementia

The assessment of the dementia is no easy task. Those who think they can diagnose or exclude or even gradually identify a schizophrenic dementia by means of an intelligence test lasting a few hours or even days must have a concept of dementia praecox that is completely different from that of the Kraepelinian school. Such investigators proceed as if all that the patient has earlier known and understood has been lost, forgetting that this form of dementia cannot be considered in a cross-sectional perspective. What we call dementia can fluctuate in time between very wide limits. External circumstances often have a decisive influence. The same patient who in the institution behaves in a completely unreasonable or demented manner can participate at home in all domestic functions and can be regarded by his relatives as healthy in every respect. The patient can show an absolute defect in logic when it comes to appreciating his own position vis-à-vis his environment. He is often quite incapable of reaching the simplest conclusion, e.g. 'If I behave in an antisocial way in the institution then they will not discharge me', even though he is daily confronted with evidence supporting this conclusion and understands the individual components of the argument as well as someone who is deemed to be healthy. He believes, however, that he has good grounds for behaving badly in so far as he is trying hard to get out of the institution. The same patient is capable, however, of presenting a well-reasoned, hour-long lecture in which he convinces most of his audience that he is of sound mind, in which he very deliberately omits everything that is contrary to his argument and embroiders, or even changes, whatever favours his theme. He can carry out complicated tasks, can show scholastic know-

ledge which his doctor might well envy, can understand that knowledge and make correct use of it. He can make refined plans for flight,
or for hoodwinking and deceiving clever people. He can at a given
moment appreciate everything that is explained to him, but an hour or
even a few seconds later he can be entirely lacking in understanding of
the very same matter. Over a given period he can furnish an excellent
account of his life history, but at a certain point he may become blocked
and seem demented. The schizophrenic, however, is no simple
dement; he is demented in respect of certain issues, certain periods of
time, or certain complexes only.

Acute stages of the disease

It is generally recognised that it is better to diagnose the dementing
process early. Unfortunately the various empirical rules which have
been put forward for achieving this are not helpful. This is probably
because there are two sets of phenomena which occur in the early
stages of the illness. One set does permit us to reach certain conclusions
about the nature and strength of the schizophrenic process, for
example certain disturbances of association, but other phenomena also
occur in other illnesses and tell us nothing about the nature of the
process or about its severity, for example manic and depressive
symptoms. Our task is therefore to look beyond these general
phenomena, seek out what is specifically schizophrenic and then
assess, according to their severity, those symptoms which we can say
with certainty or even with some degree of probability will persist.

Where the first attacks are manic or, as is more common, melancholic
in nature, it is relatively easy to distinguish the specific symptoms of
schizophrenia, namely the disturbance of association and of affect. The
more pronounced these are, the worse the prognosis, because these
are precisely the disturbances which show least improvement.
Catatonic symptoms are significant, too, since they reveal, behind the
affective fluctuations, a schizophrenic process, the seriousness of
which corresponds by and large to the overt severity of these
phenomena. We must, however, be cautious in drawing conclusions,
since as long as the illness is in its acute stage these symptoms usually
show some improvement and the significance of a depressed mood is
notoriously unreliable. It has been asserted that catatonic symptoms
occur frequently in manic-depressive illness. I have so far never
observed in this illness any symptom that could be regarded on
analysis as catatonic in the same sense as the catatonic symptoms of

schizophrenia. This may be because we have admitted exceptionally few manic-depressive patients in the last few years.

In oneiroid (dream-like) states it is important to assess the genuinely schizophrenic symptoms and to base our prognosis on them, but marked confusion and stupor are usually difficult to analyse. It is rare, however, for such syndromes to persist for long in an extreme form, and periods of greater lucidity eventually make it possible to form some judgement on the presence or absence of the characteristic schizophrenic symptoms.

Chronic stages of the disease

In chronic states a considerable improvement is always possible. A transfer of location, for example, which has proved ineffectual on a dozen occasions may on the thirteenth bring about a kind of recovery. Failure to take this into account has been the rock upon which most attempts to draw up reliable principles of prognosis have foundered. At the same time it is in fact rare for recovery to be extensive once the dementia has reached a certain point and the patient has shut himself off from the outside world. I have, however, lost touch with hardly any of our admissions of the last ten years, and when patients are transferred from clinic to institution I feel regret that the improvement that might have taken place was not achieved under our care.

Distinction between primary and secondary symptoms

In analysing the power of individual symptoms to determine outcome, I lay great weight on a distinction between the primary symptoms, which are part of the disease process, and the secondary symptoms, which arise as reactions of the ailing psyche to environmental influences and to its own strivings.

To take an analogy, it is possible for osteoporosis to reach a very advanced stage without obvious symptoms, until the patient suffers a physical trauma. The real disease, and with it the prognosis, lies in the brittleness of the bones which can, depending on external circumstances, produce symptoms or not. Further, it is not always possible to reach conclusions about the severity of the illness by relating the symptoms to the seriousness of the event that caused them: a severe trauma, for example, can break a normal bone. In osteoporosis brittleness is the primary symptom, the break resulting from a slight trauma is the secondary. Similarly an abductor paralysis is a primary symptom, while the contracture of the internus and the ocular spasms are secondary symptoms. The latter have nothing to do with the prognosis of the illness. They depend on circumstances which are external to the illness, for example on whether one or both eyes are covered.

To find analogous differences in the phenomena that manifest themselves in schizophrenia, there is already a point of reference, namely the symptoms which are triggered by external influences, for example attacks of abusive rage which are the patient's psychological reaction to external influences, even when they last a long time and begin with hallucinations. The same significance can be attached to states of altered consciousness, including the Ganser syndrome. Here it is a question of a waking dream, a dream of desire or fear, such as are also seen in hysterical patients who have encountered an emotionally disturbing event, and in others who are not demented, but whose nervous system is labile. Thus a female schizophrenic patient with hallucinations and delusions may develop false ideas about marriage, pregnancy and motherhood. This is not the illness itself, but only an inessential symptom of the illness, triggered by some external or inner emotion. Thus states of altered consciousness have a very good prognosis. Among 18 patients with this condition only one was not restored more or less to his earlier condition. There is no question here of progressive deteriorating attacks of the illness, merely random episodes.

The disease process does not actually produce the complicated symptoms which we are accustomed to see. Particular delusions or hallucinations are not generated by the process itself. The disease process can only create certain elementary psychological disturbances, on the basis of which hallucinations and delusional ideas arise, governed by the joint effect of determinant and releasing factors. It was not the disease process which made a former patient, a widow, experience lengthy and unendurable pains in her abdomen: it was the fear of being pregnant and, finally, the conviction of pregnancy after she had had sexual relations with her neighbour. Prior to this she was a latent schizophrenic, quite capable of regular employment. The pains are a reaction of the sick mind to certain emotional events and have nothing to do with the disease process and therefore with the prognosis. Similarly, the behaviour of the patients – whether they withdraw into themselves, whether they work or not, whether or not they smear excrement – does not constitute the primary symptomatology of the illness, but rather the result of several psychological processes and external influences.

The most striking support for the idea that what we call dementia is in the main a secondary symptom comes from the sudden improvement that can take place in apparently hopeless cases as a result of psychological influences. In one institution a female patient had been kept in a cell for years because she was so dangerous. When taken along to a Christmas celebration she behaved impeccably, and on Berchtold's Day she appeared complete with couplets and after a few months we were able to discharge her fit for work. She managed to maintain herself outside the institution for many years. In her case the 'dangerousness' was not the direct consequence of her cerebral disorder, but a reaction to the precautions and compulsion used in her environment. Another female patient who was undergoing a mild phase of depression developed the idea of taking her own life and kept on trying to do herself harm. All the measures were taken that are customary in such cases; the only procedure we did not try was to ignore her behaviour, since this was too dangerous. In the end she had to be strapped to her bed, with the result that the patient, realising that all attempts were now useless, gave up trying to kill herself, and after a few days was set free. Later she became well enough to be certified as fit to manage her own affairs.

I would also include affective flattening among the secondary symptoms, recognising that this view goes against the general opinion. Admittedly it is uncommon for the disturbance of affect to remit if it is very prominent in chronic cases. In certain circumstances, however – for example, if we touch upon a patient's complexes, or if schizophrenia is complicated by senile dementia – the emotional life may suddenly revive after years of comparative dormancy. I have so far never seen disturbed associated functions restored in this way.

Catatonic symptoms are regarded by most psychiatrists as primary phenomena. I do not believe that this is correct. Stereotyped speech, for example, may represent an abbreviated symbol of a loved one; if there were no loved one, then there could be no stereotypy. I would not even consider cataleptic phenomena to be primary symptoms, since psychological influences can cause them to disappear completely and to reappear. The same applies to negativism, mutism and command automatism, all of which can have various origins.

I do regard certain bodily symptoms, such as fibrillary twitchings, muscular excitability and pupillary disequilibrium, as primary symptoms worth studying in detail as direct signs of the involvement of the nervous system. Other physical symptoms are much less easy to understand. Disturbances of the vasomotor system are very complicated and their genesis can be varied. The same applies to anomalies of diet, secretion, temperature and menstruation. Oedema occurs in the early stages of the disease, and cannot be entirely attributed to idiosyncratic postures. An increase in body weight, unaccompanied by psychological improvement, distinguishes the illness from manic-depressive insanity, but an increase in deep reflexes is a feature which the illness shares with many functional and organic disorders. The same is true of sleep disturbances and headache. All these symptoms are transient, with the exception of the twitchings and the muscular and pupillary excitability. Other frequent symptoms – dry coated tongue, loss of appetite, rapid loss of weight and energy and coarse tremor – are usually regarded as signs of an intercurrent infection.

On the psychological side the most fundamental disorder appears to be a change in associations. In schizophrenia it is as if the physiological inhibitions and pathways have lost their significance. The usual paths are no longer preferred, the thread of ideas very easily becomes lost in unfamiliar and incorrect pathways. Associations are then guided by random influences, particularly by emotions, and this amounts to a partial or total loss of logical function. In the acute stage associations are broken up into little fragments, so that in spite of constant psychomotor excitement, no kind of action is possible because no thought is followed through, and because a variety of contradictory drives exist side by side and cannot be synthesised under one unitary affective or intellectual point of view.

There is, in addition, a kind of stupor and a slowing down of all mental processes which cannot be explained as arising from secondary sources. The impression made by these symptoms is that they have an organic basis. They may be linked with the severe cerebral oedema which we usually find in fatal cases of catatonia. Many catatonic attacks also present an organic appearance: they begin with loss of consciousness and convulsions and in some circumstances are even followed by slight paresis.

Confusional states call for more detailed study. Confusion is not a unitary symptom but a phenomenon which occurs in many mental disorders, once the disturbance becomes so severe that the observer is no longer able to follow the patient's thoughts. Some forms of confusion can be attributable to the primary cerebral disorder, in that they mark the progressive attacks of the illness and reflect the disorder of association. Other forms arise because the patients' various hallucinations prevent them from being in touch with reality, though closer examination usually shows some connective thread in the ideas. We have to be careful to distinguish between schizophrenic confusional states and those which occur in mania.

Stupor is another symptom that has many different roots. It can be the outward sign of several basic disturbances which severely hamper inner activity or the expression of such activity. It is a notoriously difficult phenomenon to study.

Manic and depressive mood swings occupy a very special position, their significance varying from case to case. In rare instances they give the impression of being a chance combination of manic-depressive symptoms in a schizophrenic illness. Sometimes they seem to be triggered by the schizophrenic disease process, a view which is supported by the frequency with which the manic-depressive syndrome occurs in schizophrenia in general, and in the progressive attacks in particular. A third possibility is that states of anxiety and depression take on the role of secondary symptoms, with their origin in the basic schizophrenic thought process.

Remission of individual symptoms

So far, we have established some practical, empirical rules which can guide us in predicting outcome. An experienced psychiatrist often has a 'nose' for prognosis and may make a better prediction than one which is logically deduced from these rules. Nevertheless I believe that it is helpful to know how each individual symptom tends to remit, and how this affects the general prognosis. I also believe that a knowledge of whether a symptom is primary or secondary is the most useful guide to this. A few examples of which symptoms and syndromes tend to remit will illustrate this principle.

Acute syndromes do, of course, often die away, sometimes in a way which recalls the pattern seen in infectious delirium. Mania, depression, alterations in consciousness and rage behave in this manner. Confusion and stupor are not always part of an acute syndrome, and the hallucinations and delusional ideas which may accompany confusion and the withdrawal from the external world that occurs in stupor have an inherent tendency to become chronic. Catatonic syndromes, if acute, have no particularly sinister significance; the outlook changes, however, if they persist in a state of clear consciousness.

It is rare for the disturbance of association to improve once it has become chronic, and affective flattening will persist too in most, but not all, cases. It would seem self-evident that symptoms that are determined purely psychologically should be capable of remitting. Yet in the individual case this does not necessarily happen. Even in a mentally healthy person some experiences can leave behind a small scar; religious or superstitious ideas acquired in youth can come to the fore later, even if they have for decades been overthrown by logical reasoning. In schizophrenia we hardly ever find that delusional ideas which have receded completely lose their influence on logic and emotions. They are never entirely corrected, in the way that a normal person corrects an error that is not affected by emotion. Other symptoms, too, can become stereotyped. Thus I accept the existence of what Wernicke rightly called residual symptoms, and we can never be entirely certain that purely functional psychological symptoms will recover. An ominous sign is the patient's withdrawal from the external world.

Mechanism of remission

The disease process, which as far as we know destroys only a few cerebral elements, can recede to a certain extent. The study of cerebral pathology has made us familiar with the phenomenon of 'insult', in which a damaged organ accommodates very well to changed circumstances. It may also be that a poison arising from an infection or from a metabolic change operates for a certain period of time, after which one has to deal only with the established damage.

Conditions which are triggered by emotions, for example altered states of consciousness and attacks of rage, are self-limiting because in the end every emotion exhausts itself. This applies to the mentally ill and to the mentally healthy alike. An individual weeps or storms or rages until the tears and tempers are spent.

What seems to happen is that the mental symptoms that remain when a disease process has run its course are split off from the personality. For example, delusional ideas may continue to linger in 'cured' patients without being corrected. The patient has only 'forgotten' them; when questioned directly about them, or when another attack supervenes, he summons them forth again in undiminished strength. External circumstances contribute greatly to this process of splitting. The more external stimulation the patient receives and the more capable he is of accepting such stimulation, the sooner can this splitting take place. Therein lies the value of occupation and of early discharge, which so greatly influence prognosis.

We thus see that schizophrenic dementia is capable of receding not only in respect of individual symptoms, but also as a whole. Examples of late remission in schizophrenia are no longer curiosities; one has even come to expect them. It is no longer necessary to regard late recovery from schizophrenic dementia as proof of a wrong diagnosis.

It would represent an important achievement if the intensity of the disease process could be estimated. As long as we are ignorant of its nature we can only surmise. If, for example, cerebral oedema does play a part in severe catatonia, then the effect of raised intracranial pressure would make the clinical outlook particularly severe. However, it is still unclear whether such oedema is an expression of the schizophrenic cerebral process or not. Meanwhile, we can only assume that the severity of the associative disorder or stupor is in some way related to the severity of the disease process. Similarly, there is a strong impression that catatonic phenomena and pupillary differences are particularly prominent features of severe cerebral affection.

Problems in the estimation of prognosis

A few other points concerning the difficulty in assessing prognosis should be mentioned.

First of all, there is the question of the case material itself. Only a very small proportion of all schizophrenics come under observation in our institutions, and when it comes to the individual groups of the illness we see only a selective sample. For example, patients who recover after one attack are observed only during that initial attack; chronic patients are observed only in the late stage of the disease. With regard to simple schizophrenia, only the worst, most deteriorated cases are brought to medical attention. Mild cases of schizophrenia are admitted because of an intercurrent attack of rage, forensic complications, a burst of manic excitement, a suicidal attempt, or a bout of pathological drinking. The prognosis of such different cases may be unrepresentative of the average case.

The case material observed is also very much influenced by the admission and discharge policies of an institution. Where patients are discharged early, only the very serious cases remain on the books. Where a large institution for the care of the mentally ill is available, the inhabitants of the district may become accustomed to ridding themselves even of the more mildly ill. If an institution admits only the most severe cases, then acute cases will predominate there because, as we have seen, if they do not 'recover' they tend to develop more severe end-states than patients whose course is more gradual. Moreover, such an institution will soon fill up with chronic cases. Prognostic findings from different institutions can therefore never be directly compared.

The truth of this was made clear to me by the difficulties encountered in allocating to discharged patients a favourable or unfavourable outcome. Better criteria than those which I employed should be sought. It was fairly easy simply to divide the patients into those who were socially adequate, that is to say who could live more or less independently outside the institution and maintain themselves in the community, and those who were quite demented and needed to be looked after away from their families. Patients who fell into neither of these extreme categories were put into a special group of 'moderately demented' cases. However, this rating could not be used within the institution because hardly any patients came into the first category. Instead, those who were able to do useful work and with whom it was possible to maintain social contact were deemed to have had a favourable outcome. All remaining patients were classified as actively or passively asocial.

In the course of establishing these ratings I made the interesting observation that in Neu-Rheinau the patients with a 'favourable' outcome were more severely ill than those allocated to the same category in Burghölzli or in Alt-Rheinau. As I had known most of the patients personally for years, it seemed unlikely that this was due to an error. The observation was also confirmed by the physicians in Alt-Rheinau. The explanation for this fact, I concluded, was that Neu-Rheinau was run in accordance with new ideas and, from the start, had been organised so as to be filled by patients from every quarter of the globe. Here it was possible to create a new spirit which allowed the transformation of a number of severe and chronic catatonics into good workers. This difference between different parts of the same psychiatric service is very striking.

If the degree of dementia is used as a measure of outcome, then we encounter the problem that we have no satisfactory method of quantifying this. A true measure would only apply to the severity of the basic disturbance, whereas what we call dementia has no clear connection with the basic disturbance. Further, the fluctuating performance of the schizophrenic psyche raises the question of whether there is a true end state of the condition, i.e. a stage at which the illness neither progresses further nor recedes.

Summary

Our present knowledge in regard to the progress of schizophrenia may be summed up as follows.

The mental debility which follows an acute attack, no matter of what kind, usually continues to increase for some time after the acute symptoms have subsided and then reaches a relatively stable state, with longer or shorter periods of fluctuation. It is, however, quite rare to encounter cases who do not deteriorate. Among patients who remain in the institution the most frequent symptom is a gradual increase in the degree of dementia, hardly perceptible to those who are in day-to-day contact with the patients. It is noticeable if we examine such patients after ten or more years. It manifests itself in a reduced performance capacity, a greater apathy, and in physical and mental deterioration. The decline can be caused psychologically or by a progression of the disease process. In chronic cases the illness is less likely to come to a standstill, but in my experience there is no essential difference between chronic and acute forms.

In the majority of patients, however, severe dementia can be excluded, since they maintain themselves in the outside world, and even among institutionalised patients there are some who hold their own for decades, maintaining a certain standard throughout their time in hospital.

There is therefore no doubt that, on the evidence of our present material, the disease process can come to a standstill; that this point can occur at any stage of the illness; that many patients who are apparently stable can very gradually deteriorate with the passage of time; and, finally, that progressively deteriorating attacks can keep recurring. These new attacks may take place at any time, even after decades of quiescence. The menopause seems to be a period of vulnerability, but even much later in life acute exacerbations may still occur; there is no time limit that can be established with any certainty. It has been said that an interval of three or five years between attacks constitutes a chance of lasting recovery, but I do not believe this has been proved. As far as I am aware, there are no good statistics that provide information about the frequency of new attacks in the course of subsequent years. Such statistics would have to take into account the different forms of the illness and would also have to allow for the age structure of the material studied . . .

I do not like having to complicate rather than simplify the question of the prognosis of dementia praecox, but there is nothing else I can do. Only when all these matters have been cleared up will we be able to simplify our findings and speak with authority. Progress will be made only when the research worker looks separately at each of the many factors involved and carefully evaluates their significance in the different circumstances which pertain to each case.

Karl Kleist (1879–1960)

Karl Kleist was born in Alsace and studied under the most influential neurologists of the turn of the century – Ziehen, Wernicke and Anton. He was in charge of a neurological team caring for brain-damaged soldiers during the First World War, and then became professor of neurology and psychiatry in Frankfurt and then Leipzig.

Kleist was committed to a neurological interpretation of psychiatric symptoms, always looking for comparisons between functional disorders in psychosis and a corresponding deficit in brain-damaged subjects. This extract illustrates his attempt to explain thought disorder in schizophrenia in terms of the disturbance in language and thought which occurs in aphasic subjects with recognisable brain damage.

Alogical thought disorder: an organic manifestation of the schizophrenic psychological deficit

Karl Kleist (1930)
(Zur hirnpathologischen Auffassung der schizophrenen Grundstörungen. Die alogische Denkstörung. *Schweizer Archiv für Neurologie und Psychiatrie* **26**, 99–102)

In my search for the cerebral pathology of schizophrenic disturbances I was able to isolate in 1914, from the many varieties of confused speech which one sees in that condition, several particular disturbances which could be regarded as based on cerebral pathology. In doing so I confirmed Kraepelin's hypothesis that some schizophrenic disorders of speech depend, like similar phenomena that are found in dream speech, on functional disturbances in the temporal speech area. In addition to disturbed sentence formation and paragrammatisms, we found in some patients unmistakable and sometimes literal verbal paraphasias and word amnesias, particularly in their designation of general and abstract concepts. Another of my colleagues succeeded in showing that the understanding of speech was also disturbed: in his study he demonstrated beyond doubt the sensory aphasic nature of certain schizophrenic disorders of speech. As a counterpart to these findings in schizophrenics, I was able to show that patients with brain disease and war wounds in the left temporal lobe also demonstrated the same gross speech disorders – paraphasias and word amnesias – and even the same fine defects – the characteristic word errors, formation of new words and the strange formation of sentences – that one sees in schizophrenics.

Other schizophrenic speech disorders have closer links with motor aphasia. Many catatonics, for example, use an agrammatical form of speech, similar in nature to those with focal cerebral damage, particularly in the frontal lobe.

Such schizophrenic speech disorders and the corresponding forms of aphasia found in patients with focal disorders differ only in degree. This can be explained by the fact that the cell damage that occurs in the cortex of schizophrenics is not capable of causing such gross defects as are produced by obliteration or traumatic destruction of the cortical speech centres. There is no need to implicate other functional disorders outside the speech area in order to account for the speech disorders under discussion.

Thought disorders can also lead to abnormal speech patterns, but these are of a different kind. If speech and thought disorders are concurrent, which is mostly the case, then the resultant mixture of symptoms is hard to disentangle. In my view, observers have tended to over-estimate the part played by disordered thinking in producing peculiar speech in schizophrenics. Gruhle, for example, considered them to be a consequence of various schizophrenic tendencies – playing the fool and contrariness. I have never believed that all the disordered speech in schizophrenics originates from an aphasia-like language disorder, only that such a disorder does exist in some patients.

Moreover, within schizophrenic thought disorder itself (Kraepelin's incoherent thinking and Bleuler's primary schizophrenic disturbance of association), I believe that certain forms are explicable in organic terms. The first organic variety which I isolated in schizophrenia was paralogical thought disorder. In this form subjects cannot grasp or define objects or persons, cannot make connections which are presented or named to them and cannot correctly state the true nature or significance of these items. The relevant concepts sometimes emerge in incomplete and fragmentary fashion, and beside the point. Sometimes the true concept is replaced by loosely connected ideas and frequently several different concepts that come to him are amalgamated. The patient's thoughts then by-pass the real task and it was for this reason that I spoke of paralogias.

Since interpretations and suggestions of other irrelevant matters may thus paralogically enter the patient's head, this form of thought disorder can give rise to irrational, delusional thinking. In the cases under discussion consciousness remained clear, attention was adequate and in terms of behaviour the patients were ready for action. The disorder could not therefore be explained in terms of a general lowering of psychic activity, affecting attention or consciousness. In severe cases, I was however reminded of the agnosias, particularly the finer ideational agnosia, first reported by Liepmann. I was later able to confirm this connection with the agnosias when I observed the same symptom of paralogical thought disturbance in a patient with a lesion in the left occipital lobe. Originally it had been thought that such thought disorder in patients with demonstrable pathology in the brain was a form of flight of ideas, but the excitement of thought, the disturbed attention and the pressure of talk that usually accompanies flight of ideas are absent in paralogia. It is also probable that flight of ideas are not due to cortical dysfunction, but to a lesion in the brain stem.

Paralogical thought occurs through some breakdown at a preliminary stage in the conceptual process of speech, in the same way that paraphasia occurs from a breakdown in the preliminary process of selecting words and names. It is therefore a 'sensory' disturbance of thought; and, because of an accompanying deficiency in insight, this leads to errors in all stages of thinking. It was in this sense that I spoke of a 'disturbance in thought co-ordination'.

I had already described a different type of thought disorder in schizophrenics, characterised not so much by paralogical errors as by a failure in the thinking process. At the time I regarded it as a form of inhibition in the activation of ideas. I now consider it an *alogical disturbance of thought*. It can also be seen with damage to the left forebrain, and is characterised by a lack of productivity of thought and by an incapacity to carry through a chain of thought. Such patients show poverty of thought and are incapable of producing coherent thoughts from single ideas or perceptions. They cannot draw conclusions and are unable to pick out similarities or differences when presented with several facts. The 'thought formulae' of ordinary thinking operations seem to have disappeared. It is difficult to distinguish between alogical thinking from frontal disease and defects in thinking that follow brain stem lesions, but there is no doubt that the alogical thought disorders which occur in forebrain injury match closely those that occur in schizophrenia, particularly the hebephrenic variety.

So far as the psychology of thinking is concerned, the occurrence of paralogical and alogical disturbances shows that thinking is not one simple dimension but, like speech, combines sensory and motor components. It also implies that thinking does not have a single cerebral substrate, but at least two, a system in the posterior cerebral area and one in the forebrain. There is the same relationship between 'rational thinking' (together with its pathological variety – paralogical thought disorder) and 'executive thinking' (and its pathological variety – alogical thought disorder) as there is between understanding of speech (and receptive aphasia) and the execution of speech (and expressive aphasia).

Paralogical and alogical thought disturbances do not exhaust the clinical forms and possible organic substrates of thought disorder in schizophrenics. I would not include within this framework stereotyped and reiterative disturbances in thought, perseveration, incoherence and distractibility of thought that go with inattention and excitement, or the play of foolish thoughts that doubtless originates in morbid affective states. As far as one can say at present, such disorders involve the brain stem, while it is the cortex which gives rise to paralogical and alogical disturbances of thought.

It follows that the thought and speech disturbances of schizophrenics cannot be attributed to one cause or have one common origin. Nevertheless, it is conceivable that they could all be due to some unitary and basic disturbance, such as the notions put forward by Berze (see page 52) or Carl Schneider (see page 112). The cortical speech disturbances and the cortical thought disturbances found in schizophrenics are in fact similar in kind. The simple structure of speech (the syllables and words) and the simple concepts of objects are intact, whereas higher forms of speech and the developed conceptual structures are damaged. What characterises these higher forms of speech and conceptual processes is their ability to contain references to some relationship between events, to experiences and to interpretations. It would facilitate understanding if we could reserve the term 'thought' for concepts which encompass these higher relationships, and the term 'concept' itself for ideas which have no relational content. Paralogical and alogical disturbances would then be a true thought disorder and not a conceptual disturbance.

Gustav Störring (1903–)

Gustav Störring was born in Zurich and studied medicine mainly in Bonn and Kiel. He spent most of his professional life in the academic department of neurology and psychiatry in Kiel. His articles spanned a wide range of neurological and psychiatric topics, but he was particularly interested in the alteration in consciousness which occurs in psychosis. This extract summarises his views on perplexity, a topic which is rarely discussed in the Anglo-American literature.

Perplexity

G. E. Störring (1939)

(Summary – pages 65–9 – of '*Wesen und Bedeutung des Symptoms der Ratlosigkeit bei Psychischen Erkrankungen*', Leipzig: Thieme)

In this paper I have dealt at length with the nature and significance of the symptom of perplexity ('*Ratlosigkeit*', not knowing where to turn) as it occurs in various psychiatric disturbances. I did so because I believe that this symptom is of considerable importance in the differential diagnoses of mental disorders. I began by referring to Wernicke's contribution to this problem; I then dealt with Carl Schneider's work on the significance of the symptom in the experience of thought withdrawal and his decisive comments on its occurrence in other mental illnesses.

After a critical appraisal of other definitions I defined perplexity as the oppressive awareness of one's inability to cope with a given internal or external situation, this awareness being experienced as something that cannot be explained, something that has to do with one's own self. I further pointed out that perplexity must be clearly distinguished from anxiety, though the two are frequently found together.

Turning to mental disorders I dealt first with perplexity in schizophrenia, since there is a certain quality in schizophrenic perplexity which makes the symptom to some extent pathognomonic for this illness. In contrast to Wernicke, I stated that it is not only acute mental changes of sudden onset that lead to perplexity, but that in schizophrenia, unlike organic states, a perplexed mood arises even when the illness is of gradual onset if the patient becomes aware that his empathic capacity is growing less, that his activity is declining and that he is gradually becoming detached from the world of perception. This strange turning in upon one's self, which occurs when thinking and will are experienced as outside one's control, in negativism, in obsessional states and in certain experiences of bewitchment, puts the terrified patient into a state of perplexity. Taken together with the crippling ego disturbance he has experienced, a single, unitary effect is formed with which the normal individual can no longer empathise. Such experiences are so strange that even the patients themselves cannot understand what is happening to them. This experience, which the patient cannot account for, shatters his very existence. The changes in his perceptual world perplex him because of the changes they bring to his view of this world. At the same time the strange withdrawal also bewilders him. Throughout all these experiences he is aware of an incapacity, which he cannot explain, to cope with the relevant internal or external situation.

Very often schizophrenic perplexity is associated with anxiety. Sometimes this mood change is intimately connected with the abnormal perceptual process, and has no objective correlate; sometimes it has content within his uncanny experiences. In either case it has an alien quality, which is found almost exclusively in schizophrenia, and justifies the use of the term 'anxious perplexity'.

The schizophrenic's attitude to the perplexity is also a distinguishing feature. In other psychoses a subject will treat the perplexity dispassionately, as if he were a mere spectator. In schizophrenia, it cannot be dissociated in this way, and dominates the whole perceptual world.

Perplexity usually persists in schizophrenia, whether the condition has an acute or insidious onset. This pattern contrasts with that seen in other psychoses. It is, however, hardly ever found in schizophrenics whose illness begins with delusions of persecution, and is even less common in older patients with a defect state, who have withdrawn entirely into their schizophrenic world.

The perplexity associated with manic-depressive illnesses does not have the quality of strangeness which is part of the schizophrenic experience. It also occurs much less frequently, and almost always in circumstances that are quite well defined and psychologically largely understandable. In retarded depression it is particularly rare, since here the patients identify themselves with their own disturbance in a distinctive and familiar manner. They become perplexed only when the retardation is of very sudden onset; they then see themselves confronted by urgent and difficult tasks and still maintain a capacity for thinking which is relatively good or even lively. The symptom of perplexity seems to occur more frequently in vital depressions whose onset is accompanied by depersonalisation phenomena. Considering the large number of strange experiences which such patients undergo, however, the perplexity plays a surprisingly small part. This may be because the mode of reaction is so predominantly hypochondriacal. Clinically, such cases are mostly mixed manic-depressive states of long standing, which are accompanied by many strange vital disturbances and morbid sensations, particularly in relation to the body image. In such cases there is probably also a psychopathic constitution. Perplexity occurs most frequently, and in its most richly varied forms, in very anxious mixed manic-depressive states, where the swings in anxiety and other affective phenomena lead to contradictory ideas which the patient cannot explain. In depersonalised patients of this kind a series of strange impressions occur, both internally and externally, and these, like full-blown depersonalisation, can be associated with perplexity. A state of perplexity based on the experience of being unable to maintain a consistent grasp of reality occurs much less frequently in manic-depressive illnesses than in schizophrenia or symptomatic psychoses. Anxiety in manic-depressive disorders can at times lead directly to perplexity when there is no object to which it can attach itself, so that it is experienced as something uncanny, strange and inexplicable. If the anxiety is very severe, consciousness is restricted, and this is less conducive to the development of perplexity.

As for the symptomatic psychoses, perplexity is virtually only seen when the clinical picture is one of delirium. It is based on the patient's awareness of his inability to think and act in an orderly fashion, coupled with an awareness of his inability to maintain a consistent grasp of reality. It is quite different in origin from that seen in schizophrenia, a point which can be used in the differential diagnosis of the two sets of conditions. In the symptomatic psychoses, perplexity is usually short-lived, accompanied by changes in affect, and the subject maintains some insight into what is happening. If, as in schizophrenia, there is withdrawal into the self, then one should always consider the possibility that it is not a typical symptomatic psychosis at all, but the triggering of schizophrenia by a physical condition in a predisposed individual. In chronic organic reactions, such as general paralysis and dementia, perplexity is rare. The more the organic process destroys critical faculties and affects emotional capacity, the less possibility there is of developing the symptom. In the amnesic syndrome there may often be a high degree of objective disorientation, but conditions are not usually favourable for the development of perplexity.

In reactive mental disorders perplexity is hardly ever encountered. There may be situations, even in normal psychological life, which make the individual aware of his inability to cope with them and this may be experienced as something inexplicable, something that concerns his own personality. Yet it is generally only in the very early stages of such states that this gives rise to a perplexity reaction. Usually the individual does not take long to realise that the situation can in fact be met, or it is soon dealt with in some other inner way, possibly by means of a hysterical evasive reaction or some other form of psychological reaction. Even when anxiety is pronounced in such states, the patient is always aware, with a greater or lesser degree of clarity, of the experiential basis of his anxiety. It is not inexplicable to him or experienced as alien to his personality, and therefore is seldom accompanied by perplexity. Severe terror reactions, for example, are followed by, among other phenomena, a numbness of affect or by instinctive behaviour, rather than by perplexity. In hysterical reactions the whole of the patient's experience, including the histrionic activity, reflects the innermost aims of his personality, so that here again there is no experiential reason for the appearance of perplexity. Even when the condition is psychotic rather than neurotic – a psychogenic or reactive psychosis – the patient always retains an understandable relationship with the initial affect-laden experience. Similarly, in genuine reactive depressions, the retardation and mood swings, which are responsible for perplexity in endogenous manic-depressive illnesses, are absent, and perplexity does not occur.

Hypochondriacal states are accompanied by a particular quality of emotional life, quite different from perplexity. And the alienation and depersonalisation sometimes experienced by individuals with a psychasthenic personality disorder are the consequence of a tendency to introspection, which is not conducive to the development of perplexity.

Ludwig Binswanger (1881–1966)

Ludwig Binswanger was born in Kreuzlingen in Switzerland. His father was a psychiatrist and his uncle was Otto Binswanger, whose name is associated with 'Binswanger's disease', a variety of multi-infarct dementia. He studied under Bleuler and Jung, but the main influences on his psychiatric thinking were philosophical, particularly the work of the existential philosophers, Heidegger and Husserl.

Binswanger's principal claim to attention is his attempt to interpret schizophrenia in terms of existential philosophy. Some of the trends in British psychiatry in the late 1950s and 1960s owe much to Binswanger's ideas, a point which is brought out if one scans the references in R. D. Laing's 'The Divided Self'. The following extract illustrates Binswanger's attempts to place the classical symptoms of schizophrenia within an existential framework.

Extravagance, perverseness, manneristic behaviour and schizophrenia

L. Binswanger (1956)
(Pages 188–97 of 'Drei Formen Missglückten Daseins: Verstiegenheit, Verschrobenheit, Manieriertheit'. Tübingen: M. Niemeyer)

Extravagance, perverseness and manneristic behaviour are forms of *existential failure* in the sense that an individual's sense of the flow of life has come to a stop or been frozen. At such a point, it is no longer possible for him to continue within the framework of love and friendship. This, as I intend to show in this article, is more typical of the schizophrenic's world than of a normal person's experience. These three aspects of their existential state – extravagance, perverseness and manneristic behaviour – correspond respectively in the areas of psychopathology to *rigidity, stupor* and *splitting*. For this reason the studies I have made on existential aspects of schizophrenia should help us to understand in greater depth the phenomena of splitting and stupor. I have shown in a number of detailed case histories that, whenever the flow of a person's life is threatened or arrested, that person can no longer realise himself, no longer mature, and will lose the capacity to make rapport and emotional contact with others. This arrest of the flow of existence does not mean that an individual can no longer make sense of his present world, but it does mean that his concept of a future for himself is severely impaired. One might say that the 'way to the future' is barred.

This state of affairs is illustrated in several of the cases that I have described. Ellen West was torn between an urge for gluttony and the ideal of being slim. In her own words, she saw 'all exits from the stage as barred'. In her ensuing despair she went to pieces at this stage, and the only 'exit' remaining open to her, the only way forward that she could see, lay in a decision to take her own life. In the case of Jürg Zünd, the arrest of true self-realisation took the form of seeking anonymity in the crowd. For Lola Voss the 'arrest' occurred when she abandoned herself to superstition and amateur soothsaying, prior to the development of frank delusions of persecution. In Suzanne Urban's case it was a surrender to a feeling of terror and fear.

Of the three characteristics of the existential state of a psychotic individual, extravagance appears at an early stage. It can be regarded as representing an extravagant or exaggerated concept of an ideal existence. *Perverseness*, on the other hand, is a manifestation of the contrariness of the world as it is seen, and is a preliminary stage of the schizophrenic 'arrest' of self-realisation. A normal person views the world as consisting of stable, symmetrical and natural relationships; it is a world where everything is straight, not crooked or awry. Not so the schizophrenic. For him it is contrary, distorted and disconnected: a sense of the future no longer appears natural, but is somehow unattainable and removed from the self. The connection between *manneristic behaviour* and schizophrenia is a particularly close one. It can be regarded as a 'loss of sparkle', a freezing and repetition of present existence, and a reflection of the intellectual side of man's nature rather than the 'free play' of individual life forces. It is as if there is an 'iron net' round the free expression of gestures, an invisible and incomprehensible force which is stifling the natural flow of life.

It should be pointed out that, when we talk about a 'preliminary stage' of schizophrenia, this does not mean that the characteristic triad will necessarily evolve into a florid schizophrenic illness. The existential and clinical points of view should always be kept separate. The clinical approach deals with hard *clinical facts* and the *course of an illness*. The existential analysis is concerned with unravelling what it is like to *be schizophrenic* and what it is like to change from one *mode of being to another*. For this purpose we are justified in using the language of metaphor, and to talk about the power of the 'iron net', the meaning of 'ceremony' and the role of the 'mask' and the 'grimace' in the experience of an individual. How else can we understand what it must be like to be gripped by despair and cut off from human love and trust. It was these experiences which led Ellen West to commit suicide, Jürg Zünd to seek permanent institutional care, and Lola Voss and Suzanne Urban to develop delusions of persecution.

Although I have emphasised that clinical and existential analyses should be kept separate, the existential approach can sometimes shed light on the clinical. For example, one might regard schizophrenic autism, as it is understood clinically, as a state of extreme self-sufficiency, where an individual is impervious to social influences. In fact, existential analysis has shown this to be false. It is in fact an exaggerated dependence on some aspect of the rules of society. An individual will either accept some set of rules with avid obedience, or fight against them. Either way, the nature of autism is best viewed, not as a rejection of the world of others, but either as exaggerated conformity or exaggerated opposition to it. This is clearly illustrated in the case of Jürg Zünd, who changed from being an angry fighter for society to being an extreme imitator of current social fashions.

There is one exception to the rule that schizophrenia merely causes an exaggeration of the prevailing social norms. This concerns cases of schizophrenia with a stormy onset, particularly those that begin with the 'end of the world experience' (see page 108). In such states, the 'world', as an individual knows it, disappears, and with it all the social institutions that one may live for. Even in these cases, however, the individual must rebuild his world, when the acute state is past, and he then chooses models or images which are part of his culture. This shows that schizophrenics can never 'break away' permanently from what is regarded as a 'normal' life, or achieve extraordinary artistic skills. The most that they can achieve is an extravagant, perverse and manneristic distortion of all that is typical of human existence, all that is mundane. Bleuler mentioned that one of his schizophrenic patients 'expressed trivialities in the most lofty, affected phrases, as if he were dealing with the highest interests of mankind'. Minkowski's patient (see page 201), a school-teacher who rigidly applied certain pedagogic principles without regard to whether they were appropriate, is another example of how schizophrenia desiccates and denatures existence, leaving only a shell or a mask of what life is really about.

One might say that schizophrenic existence is not only a mask of all that is real and vibrant in life, but that a schizophrenic lives behind this mask. In doing so he surrenders himself to anxiety and despair, and the world is then emptied of meaning. At an intermediate stage, when there is neither complete immersion in the normal flow of life nor complete arrest of this process, an individual may achieve, temporarily, a precarious existence. There is no sense of happiness in just being alive, however, and no capacity for love. Instead, the individual experiences a pervasive anxiety and emptiness, and looks, to an observer, as if he is numb or distracted. Later, he can no longer 'hold out' against the power of the anxiety and dread, and sinks into the abyss of a new world, warped and denuded of all the usual landmarks. The most characteristic feature of this new world which the patient has entered is its abnormal *temporal* quality. Time virtually comes to a standstill: there is no notion of a future, and the present becomes detached from its past.

Psychopathological and existential accounts of schizophrenia differ in particular on the question of what is known as *splitting*. Bleuler used the term 'split mind' to mean a loss of associative connections. His theoretical model was that of association psychology. The term is also used in psychodynamic formulations. From an existential point of view, 'splitting' means that an individual's existence is losing its personal quality and uniqueness and becoming a mere copy of some general way of life. A person loses his individuality and becomes typical of a certain class of people. The terms 'emptiness' and 'arrest' express a similar concept, the former emphasising the loss of potentiality for participation in life that ensues, and the latter the standstill in time which occurs.

To illustrate these concepts I shall now describe the case of a 39-year-old married woman, Ilse.

> Her illness and her existential change began when she put her right hand into a burning stove in order to show her father, whom she loved passionately, 'What love can do', and in order to move him by this proof of love to alter his tyrannical behaviour towards her mother. This act was indeed *extravagant*: she climbed too high. We might say that 'she went over the top'. [Binswanger's term *Verstiegenheit*, translated here as extravagance, literally means 'climbing too high', Tr.] Ilse lacked the necessary psychological experience to see that she could achieve nothing lasting by this heroic deed in the face of one as tyrannical as her father. To pursue our metaphor, an experienced 'climbing guide', someone who knew his fellow men, would have dissuaded her from such rash mental 'scaling of the heights' and would have assured her confidently that with her lack of experience in this unfamiliar and extremely difficult field, such heroic measures would get her nowhere. He would have told her that she was 'climbing much too high'.

The action may also be described as *perverse*, in that the daughter wants to make a loving approach to her father, but estranges him immediately by her choice of method. The tortured logic of her theme, namely that she will move her father and make him change his attitude and behaviour, is apparent when we consider that the action, instead of being a pure proof of love, becomes something tyrannical or violent, exercising pressure or compulsion on the father. Ilse wants to force her father to treat her mother better. 'If I take such pain upon myself', she wants to say to him clearly 'then you must treat mother better'. The rationale that equated proof of love with change of attitude on the part of her father is thus perverted into its exact opposite – into an alarming shock.

The clinical development of the case consisted in a sudden transformation of her love for her father and her sacrifice for him into acute delusions of love, reference and influence. Recovery saw a restoration of her love. The ordeal by fire, the sacrifice, was in fact the preliminary stage of a schizophrenic psychosis that lasted a year. By this I do not mean that the perverseness went on to become, in the clinical sense, a schizophrenic psychosis. I am trying to show, in existential terms, how a change took place from a world that was distorted or upside down to an actual delusional world, how an existence which was threatened by alien powers became one in which existence was overwhelmed by these powers.

Turning to the ordeal by fire viewed as *manneristic behaviour*, I should first point out that an individual who follows the traditions of his culture is not necessarily being manneristic. An artist may emulate a certain style in painting because he admires it and wants to make others acquainted with it. Ilse's behaviour, however, cannot be seen as a personal statement freely communicating her beliefs or values in this way. It was merely an act calculated to produce an effect, to appeal and even to alarm. Nor was it a freely made decision, but to a large extent carried out under the compulsion that she had to play the role of a martyr. Yet she explained to her husband, who knew of her intention, that she had to free herself of an overwhelming compulsion to carry out the ordeal by fire. What we have here is therefore a desperate attempt to play a role of her own within the confines of an existential threat caused by her fear of madness. It is this role-playing which is the essence of manneristic behaviour.

The content of her subsequent delusions support this analysis. She mentioned at this later stage that doctors were using the 'tools of martyrdom' in her treatment, that she was being exposed to the scorn and mockery of others, and that her arms were becoming cold like clay. This shows that the development of delusions can be seen as the martyr's role having, so to speak, 'got out of hand'. Whereas in the preliminary stage of the psychosis she surrenders to the mask or role while continuing to exist behind the mask, in the delusional stage it is only as a mask or a role that she does exist.

I hope that by this example I have succeeded in demonstrating the psychiatric meaning and purpose of our three concepts. I hope that I have been able to show how an existential analysis can elucidate the clinical concept of autism in terms of the flow of events that is human existence. And I hope that I have been able to explain the mechanisms whereby disturbances in this flow lead to the clinical condition known as schizophrenia. A thorough knowledge of what is happening to an individual who is overtaken by these events should help us in our practical and theoretical endeavours on their behalf.

Paul Matussek (1919–)

Paul Matussek was born in Berlin and studied theology, philosophy and psychology before turning to medicine and psychiatry. His main psychiatric training was under Kurt Schneider in Heidelberg, and he then moved to the Max-Planck-Institute in Munich. He worked briefly with H. J. Eysenck in London in the early 1950s and in 1965 he became head of the section on psychopathology and psychotherapy in the Max-Planck-Institute, where he still works.

His article illustrates the influence exerted by *Gestalt* psychology on theoretical accounts of the psychology of schizophrenia, and sheds new light on the much debated issue of delusional perception.

Studies in delusional perception
P. Matussek (1952)
(Untersuchungen über die Wahnwahrnehmung. *Archiv für Psychiatrie und Zeitschrift Neurologie* **189**, 279–318)

Introduction

A delusion is a symptom that can occur in the most diverse conditions. But while there has been a lessening of interest in its psychopathology in organic settings (e.g. General Paralysis of the Insane, encephalitis), there is still some interest in the psychopathology of delusions in the functional psychoses although, even here, the biological approach is growing in importance to the detriment of the psychopathological. This might suggest that psychopathology has little or nothing to contribute to the study of delusions, particularly with regard to differences in type which occur in various clinical conditions.

This trend, however, has implications for psychiatric research. At some future time, clinicians may be in a position to dispense with psychopathological research altogether, but at present this can only have serious consequences.

For quite apart from the clinical and diagnostic difficulties which result from inadequate psychopathological knowledge, biological research also suffers from the imprecise nature of the material it sets out to investigate. In a case quoted by Speijer, for instance, six different diagnoses were made in the course of time. Biochemical investigations, aimed at correlating such results with specific clinical entities, are of very limited value.

A classification of the psychoses, by whatever criteria, must be preceded by a more discriminating psychopathology. Such a requirement is by no means illusory. One need only recall that present-day psychopathology is still largely rooted in the views and concepts of an antiquated psychology, long since abandoned by practitioners of normal psychology because of its lack of sophistication and limited accuracy. In German-speaking countries, psychopathology is largely under the influence of the opposing concepts of 'explaining' and 'understanding' mental phenomena. In fact, the use of the criterion of 'understanding' can do no more in the case of certain psychic symptoms than lead to the conclusion that they are not amenable to understanding at all. Because of this tradition in psychopathology the interest in abnormal mental phenomena diminishes when the limits of the understandable have been reached, and the 'ununderstandable' has been defined. Not open to understanding has always meant and still means that the phenomenon can be explained only in organic terms, and no longer within a psychological framework. A primary delusion is thus regarded as an 'organic syndrome'.

Consequently, 'understanding psychopathology' strenuously resists any attempt to render understandable in psychological terms that which is 'not understandable'. Such views, inaugurated by Jaspers and still widely held today, ignore the fact that psychological investigations have their place even in the presence of primary symptoms of organic origin. Empathy must not be accepted as the sole method of psychopathology. It behoves us also to study the psychological structure of the irreducible primary symptoms, quite apart from the question of whether a symptom is amenable to empathy or not.

Loosening of the natural perceptual context

To begin with, I should like to draw attention to a change in the perceptual world of individuals undergoing primary delusional experiences. It could be described as 'the splitting of individual perceptual components from their natural context'.

Let us start with our case R. We noted that certain animals and people appeared to the patient not only as more strongly expressive of their inner nature, but also as more isolated as items of perception than would be normal. A dog, a horse and an old lady were no longer just objects among many others within a certain natural perceptual context, but specially accentuated elements against a more or less meaningless background.

It should be noted that this splitting of the conceptual context is not brought about by an increased obtrusiveness of the outward appearance of individual objects. It also occurs in the absence of significantly weighted features, and can be demonstrated when the environment is lacking in points of interest. The 'whole' of the perceptual field, however, is then seen as 'dull', 'indifferent', or characterised by some other quality.

The loosening of the natural perceptual context that frequently occurs in schizophrenia becomes clear when we compare it with perceptual relationships in normal mental life. Imagine, for instance, that on a railway station you perceive a train arriving, a group of people waiting, the station master, etc. Although you are aware of these components individually, there exists also a firm perceptual cohesion between them, formed by their co-ordination into the total perception of the railway station. That this comprehensive context is experienced directly, and as a whole, is shown by the spontaneous surprise of an observer who becomes aware of an incongruous element, such as, for instance, a writing desk on the rails.

In schizophrenia, however, the perceptual context can be more or less loosened, depending on the situation and the intensity of the acute disturbance. In the example just given, the patient would certainly perceive the train, the guard and other people, without necessarily grasping the details in their natural context. The spontaneous surprise at the desk on the rails could fail to appear given a sufficiently strong disturbance.

The natural perceptual set is here an essential precondition. In the descriptions of schizophrenic experiences, this has not received sufficient emphasis. When the schizophrenic's attention is especially invited, he too would 'know' that the desk is out of place on the rails. However, the alteration in his perceptual world so produced is not the same as his immediate reality. Furthermore, his awareness of contextual relationships, brought about by drawing his attention to such incongruous items, is at most of only limited duration. The comprehensive group images soon disintegrate again. Also, the fact that patients have to make an effort in order to comprehend the natural conceptual context confirms the loosening of the context when the set is spontaneous and not forced.

A young schizophrenic student, reporting on the early phases of his illness, had noted that particularly during 'relaxed and uninteresting moments' his experiences never gave the impression of flowing naturally:

> I was surrounded by a multitude of meaningless details. Once, in such a moment, I found myself walking to the University. When I was on the street, everything seemed as dull and uninteresting as at home. I did not see things as a whole. I only saw fragments: a few people, a dairy, a dreary house. To be quite correct, I cannot say that I did see all that, because these objects seemed altered from the usual. They did not stand together in an overall context, and I saw them as meaningless details. The way to the University also seemed to be like that. My impressions did not flow as they normally do. If I had not continuously reminded myself of where I was going, I would just as gladly have stood still somewhere.

This patient, then, was aware not only of a dull indifferent background, but also of a lack of continuity of his perceptions, both in space and over time. He saw the environment only in fragments. There was no appreciation of the whole. He saw only details against a meaningless background.

Another patient gave a similar account of the beginning of his psychosis:

> I may look at the garden, but I don't see it as I normally do. I can only concentrate on details. For instance I can lose myself in looking at a bird on a branch, but then I don't see anything else.

The rarity of such descriptions in the literature, which illustrate so clearly the loosening of the perceptual context, is due not only to the relatively small number of patients who can give an intelligent account of their own inner experiences, but also to the unobtrusiveness of the symptom. Sensory disturbances, gross thought disorder, and genuine delusional experiences are much more in the centre of experience, even for the patient himself, than the loosening of the perceptual context which is often not very marked. Even in normal subjects, such phenomena, which might appear perhaps in states of extreme fatigue, are overshadowed by more obvious changes in the overall psychic condition. For the schizophrenic patient mentioned above, it was the change in the whole atmosphere of the environment – dull, trite, uninteresting – which attracted his attention in the first instance. He might not even have noticed the contextual disturbance, if he had not found himself using a familiar route, which he had often taken before.

It should further be borne in mind that it is not a question of the context of the perceived environment being either present or absent – this context is just to a greater or lesser extent disturbed. The extent to which the context is loosened varies with the severity of the illness. It can be measured perhaps by the range of the context that is still experienced – 'range' meaning the spatial or temporal distances within which 'single elements' are still perceived as related. The more advanced the contextual dissolution the narrower does this range become.

Rigidity of perception

The dissolution of the external environment into more or less comprehensive single components corresponds to the patient's ability to lose himself in the contemplation of details. In certain states of the psychosis he can focus his attention on such isolated details for longer periods than the normal person, even when the delusional significance of the object has not yet crystallised.

Thus, one patient was continuously staring at a tree, which grew in front of the Clinic. When asked what she was seeing there, she replied: 'Nothing at all, I see the branch'. (Is that something special? I replied) 'No, no, it just gives me pleasure.' (What is it that gives you pleasure? I asked) 'Just looking at it. If I wanted to look somewhere else, I would first have to make an effort.'

Quite apart from the question of whether patients can focus their gaze on any object with equal 'pleasure', it is the ability to do so, and indeed the pleasure of doing so, which is characteristic. Looking away calls for an effort. One is immediately reminded of cataleptic rigidity, in which patients can maintain the most bizarre postures, often only for the simple reason that 'rigidity' is preferred to a change of posture.

To what extent the 'rigidity of perception' can in itself change the perception of the environment is illustrated in the following case:

> A schizophrenic patient reported after his psychosis had subsided that his attention had been attracted by the gently swinging cord of a light switch on the wall. He had failed to notice that the cord had been touched by someone else just before. 'What on earth is that?' he thought. He stared at the cord on the wall. Even when turning his head in order to look at the cord from all sides, his eyes remained fixed on the cord. And suddenly he had the impression that it was not the cord which was moving to and fro, but the wall. He then concluded that the end of the world had come.

If a normal person had gained such a dire impression, he would have corrected it by means of his other senses, which our patient however, failed to do.

The same patient reported later:

> I could have gone to the wall to confirm the veracity of my awful impressions. Instead I stayed where I was and stared spell-bound at this remarkable picture. I was not concerned to confirm the impres-

sion. I would say it was more convenient to keep looking. If I had wanted to change my position, I would have had to make an enormous effort of will.

This example emphasises how the perception of an object can change purely as a result of prolonged gazing, a process which Karl Duenker has also noted in normal subjects. For normal subjects it is in certain circumstances very difficult, if not impossible, to keep staring at isolated objects.

The schizophrenic, on the other hand, is capable, to a much greater degree, of fixing his attention on an isolated object, even if no definite delusional significance has yet been attached to it. He is 'held captive' by the object. In order to obtain an overview of the context, he would have to make an effort, and distance himself from the object, which, however, he generally finds inconvenient and tiresome. The 'element' maintains its hold on him, and will not let him go, so that even with frightening impressions, such as that of the impending end of the world, an 'objective correction' of the sensory impressions does not occur. A similar captivation by detail was noted by the author himself when he experimented with mescalin, an observation confirmed by other writers.

These phenomena had already been noted by earlier writers in the context of disturbed continuity of experience in schizophrenia. These writers had, however, interpreted them mainly in terms of disordered thinking, and had not appreciated their perceptual nature sufficiently. This neglect has its roots in the concept of perception which prevailed at the time, according to which the perceptual context was not a function of the 'elements of sensation', but rather a function of thinking. Changes in the properties of the perceived object in various contexts – changes which constantly crop up in everyday life – could not therefore be accepted as simple phenomena of perception.

If, however, 'naive experience' is acknowledged, and the psychological principles governing these events are taken into account, then psychopathology, too, will have to take note of these relationships as applicable to delusional perceptions. When the perceptual context is disturbed, individual objects acquire different properties from those which they have when the normal context prevails. The apperception of delusional significance is made possible only by the waxing and waning of those components and part elements of the normal perceptual field which make up the total perceptual picture. This, in fact, is what happens in psychosis, a process nicely illustrated in the case of R.

'Framed' perceptual qualities

Before the manifestation of gross delusional significance occurred, there appeared in the case of R. not only an emphasis on certain qualities of perception, but also a loosening of the perceptual context. These two phenomena developed in parallel. [By 'perceptual qualities' – *Wesenseigenschaft* – Matussek appears to mean the outward and changing nature of things – e.g. grimness or joy in a face, and friendliness or ferocity in an animal, Tr.] If the perceptual context had retained its normal stability, such a marked dominance of the appearance of the dog, the foal, and the old lady, would not have been possible, as the qualities inherent in these creatures as parts of a whole would have conferred a certain protection against their isolation. For the healthy subject, the dog would have been not only a lively creature personifying nature, but also 'part' of the farm, and indeed of the whole environment. A dog, after all, presents to view various qualities, depending on the context of the situation, e.g. running free, walking by the side of his master, lying at the feet of his mistress, chasing a bird, or sitting growling in front of the farm yard gate. Thus the dog which R. saw had, like the foal and the old woman, not only the features of the natural and the instinctive, but also others relevant to the total context. These qualities are normally so obtrusive that they can be ignored for any length of time only by the deliberate adoption of a certain attitude, and by concentration on a particular quality. But that which the healthy subject can achieve only through the adoption of a certain attitude is at a certain stage of schizophrenia normal and spontaneous. The schizophrenic dispenses with certain contexts and relationships. R.'s description thus becomes understandable:

> At ordinary times I might have taken pleasure in watching the dog, but would never have been so captivated by it. I would merely have thought about it later.

The inability to break away from certain objects in the field of perception thus depends not only on the enhanced obtrusiveness of the appearance of things, but also on the loosening of the natural perceptual context, which develops in parallel. Dog, foal and old woman are lifted out of the remainder of the context, and thus acquire a certain 'weighting'. They become, as it were, 'framed'. The expression 'framed' is more than an image if it is considered that pictures are normally framed, i.e. taken out of their environment. A framed picture has more symbolic content than an unframed one. The 'frame' also lends a certain protection to the significance of the perception and to its weighting. Torn from its context the perceptual content encourages delusional meaning, senseless as it may appear. It is, perceptually at least, more durable than normal perceptual context.

This, in my opinion, is one of the reasons for the firmness and incorrigibility of the delusional content. Thus, the healthy observer gains the impression that schizophrenics are talking not so much about the real character of the person or object, but rather about some superficial aspect, as has been well described by Zutt. But we are now in a position to say that this is due to the isolation of certain perceptual features, and not merely an inability to perceive these qualitative aspects correctly.

Elaboration of a new context

When the perceptual context in some schizophrenic illnesses, certainly in those with primary delusional perceptions, is disturbed, then the question arises whether other contextual relationships may be formed. Consider the following account by a patient of Beringer and Mayer-Gross:

> One is much clearer about the relatedness of things, because one can overlook the factuality of things. They don't exist, so one has nothing to do with them.

Thus, when a new perceptual context is formed, as this patient put it, 'when one is much clearer about the relatedness of things', it does not happen on the basis of the intrinsic nature of things. What, then, are the factors by which such a new context *is* formed?

We have already shown how certain aspects of things stand out by virtue of the subjective change in the perceived environment. The vividness of this outward appearance of things could, therefore, provide the substrate upon which a new morbid context crystallises. This assumption seems to be confirmed by R., when he says:

> Out of these perceptions came the absolute awareness that my ability to see connections had been multiplied many times over.

The perceptions which proved this increase in his ability to form connections were those of the dog, the foal and the old woman. In the case of the dog, he perceived it in a certain changed fashion, but this perceptual alteration diminished over time until the moment when he encountered the very same change in his perception of the young foal, namely a natural and untamed quality. In both perceptions, a context was formed. Dog and foal were for him not just two objects accidentally appearing in sequence, having accidentally similar qualities, but the expression of a more profound meaning, namely that the whole landscape and environment was rooted in nature and primordial in character, dog and foal providing two visible proofs. The patient experienced this in the form of increased ability to make connections.

The patient then became aware of the names of places in the neighbourhood, such as Erding and Freising (which contain the roots of the German words for 'earth' and 'free'). This also struck him as a link with primordial and nature-rooted matters. The context is further reinforced by his encounter with the old woman, where again a similar perceptual change was experienced. This seemed at first sight strange, all the more so because the natural and primordial originally made itself felt in young creatures, such as the dog and the foal. Although an old person can certainly embody earthy qualities, they generally have many other more obvious characteristics. The patient was completely unaware of the wealth and nature of these characteristics, although at that very moment he considered himself to be in possession of special powers of understanding the world. Indeed, according to his own admission, it would normally take him a long time, when well, to divine the character of another person, and then only incompletely; he now considered himself specially blessed with powers of insight. In spite of this, he failed at this moment to appreciate the character of the old woman in depth, and saw only what he had already seen in the other creatures.

By dint of noticing specific properties, torn from their natural context, R. entered a delusional world. When the encounter with the old woman caused him to ponder the natural qualities of this countryside, his thoughts turned more and more to his homeland of Silesia, which has similar qualities. The memory came to him of a characteristic scene from his childhood, when he had recited the poem 'The Casting of the Bell in Breslau' within his family circle. While he was still thinking about this, he suddenly found himself standing in front of a bell foundry. From then on he had the impression that he was in Silesia, and no longer in Bavaria, or more accurately he no longer knew where he was, Silesia or Bavaria. The impression was so compelling that he had to ask himself: 'Are my senses deceived, or is it really true that I am in Silesia?'

Here, too, we note the selectivity of perception against the background of previous experiences. While at first he only perceived the natural and primordial, which reminded him of his homeland which had similar qualities, he now suddenly sees a piece of his homeland.

His experience is not the observation of a similarity, but rather a direct physical impression, almost amounting to a sensory illusion. In order to understand this psychologically, I should now like to consider in greater depth what is known as 'symbolic context'. It is generally assumed that in these cases one is dealing with the experience of a symbolic relationship: the reality, in this case, being the bell foundry, and the symbol the homeland.

Symbolic context and identification on the basis of similar qualities

Gruhle considered that the connection between a perceived object and its abnormal significance was a delusional and specific symbolic relationship. He thus considered delusional significance to be an elaborated mental phenomenon and not one that was immediately experienced. Storch took issue with this point of view, and pointed out that in characterising schizophrenic experience, expressions like 'symbol' and 'metaphor' have to be used with the greatest caution, and should not be equated with the meaning that the word symbol has in normal psychology. In schizophrenic thinking, the images do not merely have a representational function. In fact, awareness of a substitute or replacement of a thought with an image, or awareness of straightforward equivalence might be entirely lacking. Kurt Schneider argued along similar lines, and more recently Gerhardt Schmidt rejected the characterisation of delusion as an abnormal symbolic awareness.

These views also express the point that I should like to make regarding the contrast between reality directly encountered and reality realised in the mind. Abnormal significance is perceptually encountered as an integral part of the object. It is not primarily deduced, thought out, or dredged up in some other way from our thoughts, but rather experienced directly as inherent in the object. Storch has described this phenomenon at length, but was reluctant in the end to attribute it specifically to perceptual disorder. However, without the assumption of a disturbance of perception it would be impossible for the patient to report with such conviction that he had experienced a delusional meaning so directly. Hedenberg, Otto Kant and others, who have devoted themselves to the problem of delusional reality, consider that the criterion which distinguishes a genuine from a non-schizophrenic delusion is the very quality of its being sensed, experienced and encountered. The schizophrenic who experiences the meaning of 'innocence' in the white bark of a birch tree does not 'perceive' the colour of the bark as a symbol of innocence, but sees incorporated in the white bark a very definite quality, namely that of innocence.

Changes in perception can, however, be less marked, once the relationship between the object and its abnormal quality has become fixed. Initially, however, in primary delusional perception, the object is experienced in a different way from that which applies later. For this reason, the patient just mentioned specifically denied having experienced a symbolic context:

> If I had merely meant that, like one says white is the colour of innocence, then the tree would not have had that effect on me.

The reason given by the patient for rejecting a symbolic context as characteristic of a delusion is very revealing. The effectiveness of the inner meaning, the perceived appearance of the object, distinguishes the delusional experience from symbolisation in normal mental life, even though this may not be the only difference, as we will demonstrate below. But if the qualitative aspects and the contextual relationships of perceptions are so important in the experience of significance, then certain experiences of symbolism can also be reduced to one perceptual quality that is common to two different situations, things or persons. This was noted by Conrad in a different context.

Such identification, based on similar qualities, is found in normal mental life, particularly in children and primitive people. The parallel between schizophrenic mental life and that of children and primitive people was emphasised by Storch and Schilder. Children react preferentially to the outward appearance of faces (e.g. friendly, cross, grim) while the more intrinsic features of things, such as texture or shape, are perceived to a much lesser extent. Metzger recalls, for example, how in his first years at school the figure 3 appeared to him on different occasions as proud, humble, cheerful, tired, and once even as stuffed up with cold. The actual significance of the figure receded behind the web of these qualitative impressions. In later years, this ability is gradually lost. The same developmental feature was found by Metzger among primitive people. He described an African tribe who had 80 words to convey the character of a person's gait, as it was affected by the mood, height and posture of the person. Civilised man uses only perhaps a quarter of these, because he is less able to perceive the varied features expressed in individual gait. Primitive man also uses the same word for things which to us have little in common, but to them resemble one another in respect of some shared quality. For example, an umbrella and a bat share the same word (Werner). The opening of an umbrella and the spreading of the wings of a bat suggest the same outward appearance.

This peculiarity of perception is important for the so-called 'phenomenon of identification', as seen in schizophrenia as well as in primitive mental life. Lévy-Bruehl, Werner and Storch propose that this phenomenon is a form of thought disorder. In my view, it is better regarded as a change in the *Gestalt* structure of the perceptual world, in which certain qualitative aspects predominate. In such a world a totem animal is identical to a person, because they share certain features. In schizophrenia, too, there may be misidentification of people, documented by Scheid and Conrad, and shown to be examples of delusional perception. Two people who resemble one another in respect of one characteristic are experienced as identical, a phenomenon which incidentally also occurs in mescaline intoxication. R.'s experience, described above, that he was wandering in his Silesian homeland becomes understandable in the light of these observations. The surrounding countryside became for him his Silesian homeland, because both landscapes, one in his immediate perception and one in his memory, had shared features.

Other disorders of significance in schizophrenia

Schizophrenic patients not only produce the kind of experience of significance which has just been described, but exhibit a variety which has its roots more in imagination and thinking than in perception. They are more closely related to obsessions than to delusions. For these phenomena the term 'symbolic awareness' or 'symbolic experience' is more appropriate. To illustrate this, consider the description given by a 31-year-old schizophrenic:

> We were drying the dishes and we already had quite a heap. I said, without thinking anything in particular, 'Let's make another heap.' Almost immediately this took the meaning of a heap of muck. The other day someone said that in this café they danced in the open air. Immediately I'd heard the word, no even before it had actually been spoken, I noticed that it meant something, namely that they danced here in the nude. When I hear people mention blood, it always means menstrual blood, just as the bonnet of a car always means the protective sheath of sexual intercourse. The other day one of the older farmers was addressed as 'father'; immediately it went through my mind that I was his son. I always experience such meanings with words like that; they come at me directly. With new words there is usually a little time before the meaning becomes apparent.

The abnormal meanings here do not arise from changes in perception, such as a predominance of certain qualities of things. Rather, they arise from a need to interpret the meaning of events in a compulsive manner. The patient observed that he was 'compelled to give things a second meaning, especially if they were words spoken by other people'. This demonstrates that we are not dealing with playful interpretations or with a change in the perception of an object, but rather with a 'compulsive' mechanism generated from within.

This compulsive experience is usually recognised as foreign and not part of a subject's real self, unlike delusional perception which *is* regarded by a subject as part of himself. This point, ignored by most writers on psychopathology, is further evidence of the perceptual basis of delusional perception. The two disorders of significance – compulsive and perceptual – also differ in their consequences for the subject. In the latter, a subject will complain about the content of the ensuing delusion (e.g. complain of being persecuted); in the former he will complain only that he is compelled to find new meanings.

In the compulsive variety, the abnormal significance is appreciated not as an integral part of the object, but only as connected with it. The meaning it has for the subject is not an external reality, encountered along with the object, but more an 'inner', imagined reality, transferred to the object as it were compulsively. In fact, Kurt Schneider's view that there are two stages in the development of a delusional perception – normal perception, then delusional significance – is, in my view, wrong. Delusional perception has only one stage. He appears to have been referring to these other compulsive disorders of significance, which do proceed in this manner.

A further difference between compulsive and perceptual disorders of significance is that in the former the derived meaning is rarely unshakable. It is more in the nature of an assumption, opinion or fantasy about an object than a direct experience of some significance being attached to the object.

The essential difference between these two types of disorder becomes even clearer when one contrasts the compulsive disorder of significance as seen in obsessional neurosis with true delusional perception. In the former case, according to von Gebsattel, the subject's world has an imaginative, fictitious and subjective character, in contrast to that of a primitive man or a schizophrenic. The way an obsessional patient encounters the world is no different, in essence, from how a normal person thinks about the world.

The following hypothetical case illustrates some of these points. A patient with acute schizophrenia observes a 'persecutor' wearing an overcoat. A few moments later he discovers an identical or similar overcoat worn by another person. The second person can then under certain circumstances also be perceived as an enemy. According to our hypothesis, the overcoat is here perceived as possessing the quality of hostility, with the result that both people are experienced as identical in their nature. The appearance of the overcoat is the critical factor in this process. An obsessional patient, on the other hand, would not experience anything very remarkable in the events just described. If, however, he regarded the overcoat as infected, he would avoid the second person only if his coat were *exactly* the same as that of the first person, and not just similar, or if the two coats had been in contact. For him, it would be irrelevant whether he had seen the contact or only heard about it. What matters is not the appearance of an event but knowing about it. In summary, one might say that in an acute delusional illness the significance is based on what is heard and seen, rather than what is known; in an obsessional subject, the abnormal significance is inspired by what he knows, not by what he perceives.

This explains why many obsessionals know in advance of a perception that the experience to come will have a meaning beyond its inherent significance. In cases of acute delusional illness, on the other hand, the impression of significance never appears until it makes itself manifest in the perceptual field. In such cases the experience of significance may only have a vague content: the patient knows that the object has a different significance but not what this new significance is. Here too the impression of vague significance is governed by the object itself. It is the very uncertainty regarding content, combined with unequivocal certainty of a change in significance, which demonstrates the intimate relationship between delusional perception and perceptual disorder. If it were otherwise, the patient would be content with any old meaning and would not struggle to find the real meaning.

In conclusion, it would appear justified to reserve the term 'primary delusional perception' for an experience in which changes in perception can be demonstrated, and to suggest the term 'symbolic awareness' for experiences of significance which are based on 'knowing'.

Summary

1. Delusional perception, an important symptom of schizophrenia, cannot be structurally defined within the framework of traditional psychology. In this article I have chosen *Gestalt* Psychology as a frame of reference.

2. In schizophrenics with clear-cut delusional perception, there is an over-emphasis and a widening of certain qualitative features of things, a process which may occur before delusions appear. This allows us to explain certain phenomena of delusional states, which so far have remained inexplicable. The phenomena which now become clearer include the predominance of certain perceptual qualities over other properties of objects in the world and the intrusiveness of the experienced significance, even in cases in which a delusional content has not yet become manifest.

3. In the same patients there is an associated loosening, or dissolution, of the natural perceptual context and a morbid capacity for fixing on certain details of the perceptual field. Certain components of the field are 'framed', which lends protection and emphasis to the abnormal meaning.

4. In many deluded patients, the new perceptual context is formed, not of concrete, but of more abstract properties of the perceptual world.

5. Delusional misidentification, previously considered a consequence of symbolic association, is not usually derived in this way, but stems rather from the false identification of two objects on the basis of shared qualities.

6. This disorder of significance (primary delusional perception) can be clearly differentiated from a disorder of significance which has more in common with obsessions. These can also occur in schizophrenia, although they are more common in obsessional neurosis. We suggest the term 'symbolic awareness' for this other disorder. In delusional perception, the underlying disorder is one of perception, while in symbolic awareness it is one of 'knowing'.

Gerhardt Schmidt (1904–)

Gerhardt Schmidt trained in Frankfurt and in Munich, where he worked with Kurt Schneider. His principal position, which he held from 1947 until his retirement in 1974, was as consultant psychiatrist in Lubeck, in North Germany.

He was not a prolific writer on psychiatric topics but the following article is a comprehensive review of German ideas on the nature of delusion, covering the 'Golden Years' of German psychiatry.

A review of the German literature on delusion between 1914 and 1939

G. Schmidt (1940)

(Der Wahn im deutschsprachigen Schrifttum der letzten 25 Jahre (1914–1939). *Zentralblatt für die gesamte Neurologie und Psychiatrie* **97**, 113–43)

Introduction

This survey, which covers the German literature in the 25 years up to 1939, deals with delusion as such rather than with delusional illness. A survey such as this does not seek to be comprehensive. Our main concern has been to cover all that is new in the publications on the subject of delusion over the last 25 years.

Modern psychiatry is divided into two camps, one primarily concerned with the description of morbid phenomena, the other with their genesis. Our presentation will likewise fall into two parts. In the first of these a disproportionate amount of space is devoted to a review of phenomenological and functional approaches to delusion. The amount of space taken up in this way may seem excessive relative to the number of publications involved, but this is due to the fact that we are dealing with a completely new direction in research, initiated by Jaspers, which explores the existence rather than the nature of delusion (its 'being there' rather than its 'being so'). In the second part we touch briefly on attempts to make delusion understandable in the context of normal mental life, for instance its relationship to belief and error. But these notions are of less interest than a discussion of the psychological essence of delusion and, for this reason, more space is given to those writers who have attempted to unravel the threads which lead from a normal personality to a morbidly deluded one.

Part 1a – Descriptive studies of primary delusion

Phenomenological approach
Jaspers brought order into the chaos of what was previously described as delusion by first distinguishing, according to psychological criteria, two classes of delusional ideas:

> Some can be understood in the light of related affect, other experiences, hallucinations . . . others are not amenable to further psychological analysis but are phenomenologically irreducible. The former we call delusion-like ideas, the latter genuine delusional ideas . . . We would describe as genuine delusional ideas only those which have their manifest source in a primary pathological experience, or can be explained only in terms of a personality change.

Genuine delusional ideas are in many cases experienced with immediate clarity, but may also be heralded by primary delusional experiences, such as a delusional mood state (delusional atmosphere). The question which then arises is how far the judgement 'expressed' in the delusional idea is appropriate to the original experience, how far it is fortuitous, and how far it is symbolic in the psycho-analytical sense of Freud. Having made the fundamental distinction between delusion-like and genuine delusional ideas, Jaspers further subdivides the latter into delusional perception, sudden delusional ideas, and delusional awareness. In *delusional perception* there is an immediately experienced change in a particular perception, though the perception itself remains completely unaltered from the sensory point of view. There is on the one hand a delusional interpretation in which objects and processes, that is to say the contents of a perception, suddenly acquire a new but not clearly defined meaning. On the other hand there is a delusion of reference, when the content of the perception is experienced as being significantly related to the person of the patient. *Sudden delusional ideas* can be illustrated by the example of a patient who is suddenly overcome by the conviction that there is a fire in the neighbouring town and sees it all in great detail. They appear as sudden notions, new aspects and new meanings of remembered life experiences. *Delusional awareness* is knowledge of events without clear sensory perception.

Jaspers' findings were later elaborated by Gruhle, who urged that delusion had to be viewed phenomenologically and that Jaspers' concept of morbid or faulty self-reference was too narrow; it ignored the existence, according to Gruhle, of delusional ideas which are not related to the self. A sudden, irreducible and unmotivated experience of self-reference is, however, undoubtedly the commonest form of genuine delusion and must be regarded as a primary symptom of schizophrenia. Gruhle did not regard it as pathognomonic of schizophrenia, as he later described it in epilepsy and toxic states. According to his early views, set out in 1915, the essence of the abnormality was the delusional activity itself, which was not yet associated with any specific content:

> It is just those cases, in which the patient knows that there is a meaning but not what that meaning is, which illustrate the primary nature of this morbid happening.

The development of a genuine delusion, one lacking both external cause and inner motivation, is regarded as the 'establishment of a relationship without cause'. The deluded patient is quite unable to account for what it is that strikes him as unusual in his environment. The pointless accounts given by these patients demonstrate again and again that something quite banal is suddenly imbued with significance, often with an unpleasant tone. This:

> something is never definable, as it is hidden between and behind objects and their interrelationships; it lies in the symbol.

The relationship created by the delusion is a symbolic one. But why only certain events are experienced as significant, why one is accepted in a straightforward manner while another is understood symbolically – this remains a mystery. The element of strangeness in the content of perception lies solely in its abnormal significance.

> The patient is not disturbed in the so-called elementary components of his perceptual experience (colour, etc.), nor in their shape and form (the object has this particular shape), nor in their functional meaning (this is a table), nor in his further intellectual elaboration (this is a rococo table), but only in the compulsion of his symbolic experience (this table means that the whole world is as twisted as its legs).

Perceptual change comes only with the delusional experience. The delusional experience does not, however, arise from a disturbance of perception. An apparent exception to this rule is the so-called 'end of the world experience'. In such cases it only seems that the delusional atmosphere alters the quality of perception – in fact such cases are quite different from those in which the anxious patient, because of his anxiety, misinterprets much of what is going on. Wetzel, however, who in principle takes the same view, concedes that genuine changes in perception can occur. Mayer-Gross, moreover, sees no reason why the immediate experience of significance should not be associated with pathologically altered perception. As a general rule, however, as Gruhle puts it, the act of perception and the symbolism are two different things altogether. Just as it is quite consistent for a black, red and gold ribbon to be merely a ribbon on one occasion and a political symbol on another, so it is equally possible for the paranoid schizophrenic to walk behind his plough, believing himself to be the saviour of the world. The symbolic experience facilitates the double orientation. Thus when Gruhle characterised the act of delusional perception as the 'establishment of relationship without cause', he does not deny the existence of delusional ideas without reference – primary beliefs in relationships or values, or delusional awareness – although he regards these as extremely rare. Later, he had to concede that delusional ideas could exist in their own right without being attached symbolically to an object, and concluded therefore 'that the essence of the delusional idea does not lie in the idea itself'.

Elaborating these notions of Jaspers and Gruhle, Kurt Schneider tried to define the essence of delusion even more precisely. According to him, delusional perceptions do not depend directly on the delusional atmosphere from which they often develop:

> At best they are embedded in it, but not derived from it. In no way does the specific content of the delusional perception follow from the delusional atmosphere, which is vague and has a neutral content. Not even in its emotional colouring does the delusional atmosphere have to agree with the concrete delusional perception.

The primary delusional perception belongs to those experiences, described by Gruhle as qualitatively abnormal, which lie beyond the limits of normal reactive experience and which as first rank symptoms are pathognomonic of psychosis, generally schizophrenia. Occasionally they occur also in alcoholic psychoses, epileptic twilight states, organic cerebral disorders and symptomatic psychoses.

The very rare delusional ideas which take the form of memories and imaginings, as well as the vastly more common cases of delusional awareness – knowing without sensory imagery – are included in the concept of the sudden delusional idea. For the rest, the more abstract notions, such as ideas of persecution, ancestry or special vocation, are often associated with delusional perceptions. So far as the sudden delusional idea is concerned, there is no characteristic form of experience and no particular psychological structure. This poses a major problem in elucidating the nature of delusion. While delusional perception proceeds, as it were, in two phases – first there is a particular perception, then it acquires a particular meaning – the criterion of acquired significance is lacking in the single-phase sudden delusional idea. It is conceivable that biphasic delusional ideas could occur in the same way as delusional perceptions, i.e. sudden notions associated with an abnormal awareness of significance, but this is not relevant to the problem. The sudden delusional idea lacks the positive characteristics of a delusion and thus lacks the only valid phenomenological feature which differentiates it from other ideas, including over-valued and obsessional ideas. This lack of a function of its own is important, because the only remaining criterion, that of an origin without cause – the absence of any relationship with the personality – is not always enough. Other sudden notions too can at times be more or less obviously primary, so that in differential diagnosis one would have to resort to aspects outside the delusion itself, such as the degree of improbability and other symptoms that accompany psychotic states. To demonstrate the awkwardness of using criteria derived from content, Schneider writes:

> A sudden idea could be feasible and yet be delusional, while a delusional idea might appear to be impossible and yet be true in reality.

Schneider includes sudden delusional ideas among his 'second rank symptoms'. For Schneider the basic form of delusion consists of delusional perception, which is always serious and weighty, and sudden delusional ideas, which are often playful. He talks of delusional ideas when the patient firmly believes in the reality of these experiences and elaborates their contents. In the end it is no longer possible to distinguish primary delusional experiences from secondary delusional elaborations. The word 'idea' is incidentally used in its colloquial sense, and thus includes judgements. There is therefore no need to introduce the concept of 'delusional judgement'.

Once content has been discarded, the task of analysing what is concealed psychopathologically behind delusional ideas and complex delusional experiences is by no means easy. Speaking of the schizophrenic's 'end of the world' experience, Wetzel (1922) pointed out that it can appear as a primary experience of significance or as a delusional awareness, but also as the ultimate 'realisation' of a sinister mood state that cannot be compared with any other experience. In cases where a particular form of mood and feeling permits the patient to experience the impending catastrophe 'as if' the world were about to end, in other words when the patient remains fully aware of the symbolic nature of the experience, we are still within the realm of empathy and understanding. As a primary delusion, however, it lies outside the limit of the psychology of understanding. Obviously the patient must have known about the 'end of the world' before, otherwise it could not have become the content of the delusion. Wetzel did not accept that the content – the end of the world – had been randomly selected from available material. He believed that in schizophrenia the precise content represents something very special, consistent, in this case, with a preoccupation with cosmic events and grand relationships. Delusions of the impending end of the world are generally preceded by the classical delusional mood of euphoria, dysphoria or a mixture of the two. Wetzel cannot adequately explain the special relationship that clearly exists between the theme of the end of the world as content of delusional thinking and certain affective states in schizophrenia. He suggests that quantitatively, and perhaps also qualitatively, abnormal feelings of happiness and redemption tend to become rapidly attached to something concrete, in this case the end of the world, as a transition to something newer and grander. The end of the world emerges from an atmosphere of impending doom – it is an experience of horror and destruction arising from a background of altered feelings, agonised perplexity, a sinister sense of dread, and a frightening awareness of being at the very centre of these happenings. Superficially similar experiences may occur in manic-depressive states but they are in effect different in nature: they are symbolic comparisons, expressing not so much a terror of impending cosmic catastrophe but a horror of existence itself and of the end of being. The end of the world experience that is found in epileptic twilight states, on the other hand, in so far as it derives from the threatening character of epileptic sensory disturbances, should not be considered a primary delusion.

Misidentification, especially of people, is a further example of the phenomenological multiplicity which underlies delusional experiences. Gruhle speaks of delusional misidentification as symbolic delusion or double orientation. Strictly speaking, of course, these are not genuine misidentifications. Scheid (1937) considers that misidentification of persons can be a delusional perception, sudden delusional idea or delusion-like thinking. Misidentifications of a playful kind, in the absence of dementia, should always be regarded as sudden delusional ideas. The delusional attribution of past roles to people who are identified perfectly correctly and unambiguously in the present, however, should not be included in the concept of personal misidentification. The delusion in such cases can be interpreted as sudden delusional ideas or as the 'establishment of a relationship without cause'. If

Gruhle regards schizophrenic memory distortions and the experience of *déjà vu* as an experience of reference, 'self-reference without cause', then this can be valid only in the absence of the normal insight associated with ordinary *déjà vu* experiences. But even in cases of this kind it seems to us that one is dealing less often with delusional perceptions pregnant with meaning than with a sudden delusional idea appearing in a particular set of circumstances and coupled with the certainty that all this has happened before. The realm of sudden delusional ideas includes the so-called back-dating of delusional content, as when the schizophrenic patient has the delusional idea that his present delusional idea had already occurred to him years ago. One can also agree with Gruhle that in these cases the quality of familiarity is an attribute of the delusional idea. This is not the same as when otherwise clear and undistorted memories acquire, in Gruhle's sense, immediate significance deriving from nowhere. The many different ways in which the phenomena of *déjà vu* and memory distortions can be interpreted have been discussed by Gruhle.

Kolle (1931) has studied the delusional systems of paranoid patients extensively. His work highlights the importance of the concept of genuine delusion in differential diagnosis and in the delimitation of psychopathic delusional states. Kolle investigated 66 cases which fitted into the definition of paranoia as propounded by Kraepelin, Lange and Kehrer. Of these, 62 showed the establishment of a relationship without cause, while in the remaining four he assumed the presence of a primary delusion, in view of the absence of an 'explanation by motive' (Binswanger). The demonstration of psychological irreducibility was made easier by his use of Binswanger's formulation (for example, by showing it was impossible to explain the delusion of jealousy in terms of motive), rather than the semantically ambiguous concept of understanding. In particular Kolle explored the occurrence of delusion from the functional point of view rather than from that of content, and found, on applying Gruhle's criteria (egocentric/non-egocentric, explicit/inexplicit, well-formed/formless, affectively coloured/without affect), that the main characteristics of a delusion were its well-formed nature and its unpleasant affective colouring; it was noteworthy that affect was absent in only one case.

Among foreign writers represented in the German literature, Westerterp (1924) uses examples of persecutory delusions occurring in pure paranoia to demonstrate the primary and process nature of delusion in general. For him the sole primary phenomenon is that:

> the purpose and meaning of an object, which in normal people is

conveyed directly and correctly in its perception, is in deluded subjects judged incorrectly.

This definition is rather trivial, and Westerterp regards as insoluble the question of whether the essence of a delusion is a primary affective disturbance with another 'vision' of the environment, or a selective change in perception. He therefore contents himself with the statement that, during this initial 'phase of uncertainty' (as he describes the delusional mood state), the primary element in the patient's affect is in every case his altered attitude to the environment.

The irreducibility of a primary delusion is analysed in a most individual way by Hedenberg (1927). According to him:

> the typical schizophrenic delusional idea has the character of some-
> thing that is given. It is experienced by the patient with the immediacy
> of a sensation . . . It arrives out of the blue; suddenly and with
> certainty it is there.

It derives from the schizophrenic's feeling of passivity, unrelated to desires and experience, as a given reality within the primary delusional experience. Delusion experienced as reality is the main theme of the investigations of Hedenberg, who was influenced by Lipp. He considers that the subjective reality of the deluded patient, which only by accident coincides with common reality, is in its power of conviction comparable to religious belief – there can be no question at all of contradiction or of impossibility. Bound as we are to view the world as a synthetic whole, it is impossible for us to understand this experience, which needs no connection with the existence of the individual and plays itself out in a new reality of unrelated components.

Von Domarus (1929) takes a view not unlike Gruhle's when he contends that 'delusion is distorted meaning'. To von Domarus a delusion is present when professed meaning or significance occurs within ideational reality, that is to say, reality which acquires meaning from the thinking of the individual. We will content ourselves with this sketchy outline of the author's views as they are rather poorly formulated.

Zutt (1929) also agrees with Gruhle that in a delusion things suddenly, and without recognisable cause, acquire a particular meaning, He differs, however, from the authors so far mentioned in that he examines the actual process-like personality change which all writers on the subject assume to occur, and attempts to demonstrate a direct connection between this and the delusional events. He traces the primary delusional experience back to this personality change, which he regards as its inner cause. What he means by this can be illustrated by considering an actor, who adopts a different character in the course of a play, but then reverts to his true self at the end of the evening. If, by some chance, he did not revert back to his normal personality, and was unaware that he was still his stage personality, the world around him would itself appear the focus of the change – he would be deluded. In the case of a patient who is undergoing a personality change such as Zutt describes, his environment too will be reinterpreted according to the new rules that his new personality and 'inner attitude' require. At the onset, while he still retains some insight into the change within him, Bleuler's so-called 'double book-keeping' is to be found. Two separate styles of interpreting the world will exist side by side, a state which may be compared with the playful interpretations indulged in by some normal subjects who enjoy mimicry and impersonation. At a later stage the healthy personality identifies with the morbid inner attitude (in spite of the schizophrenic discord between them), as a result of which the patients surrender completely to their delusions.

Heveroch (1919) sees in delusions of reference a clear 'disturbance of the self, or self-ness'. Delusions of reference are for him a pathological alteration in the awareness of causality, according to which patients perceive a causal or final nexus where it does not exist. But awareness of causality, which is independent of thinking, feeling and will, is a function of our whole being, and delusions of reference must clearly involve a morbid disturbance of the self, or self-ness. Whatever one might be inclined to say in response to speculations of this kind, Berze's reply that one should look for the disturbance in some specific mental function brings us back to the central problem of delusion.

The analysis of mental functions

Carl Schneider agrees with Jaspers' view that a delusion is basically incomprehensible, but regards Jaspers' notion that it is phenomenologically irreducible as incorrect, because it may form a complex of largely understandable content contaminated by bizarre content derived from certain psychotic experiences. He distinguished the following parameters by which a delusion could be evaluated: plausibility of content, the degree of certainty attached to the experience, its importance to the patient, the degree to which the content is related to life experiences and finally the manner in which the delusional thinking is carried out [the presence or absence of what we now call formal thought disorder, Tr]. Carl Schneider was concerned almost exclusively with formal thought disorder, and ignored the fact that the delusions which occur in non-schizophrenic mental illnesses must develop in a different way. In schizophrenia, according to him, delusions were a manifestation of a single pervasive change in thought processes which was the primary cause of all schizophrenic phenomena. They might arise because faulty connections would be made between different external impressions, or between external impressions and the patient's present circumstances, or because perceptions would be related to thoughts which happen to be present, or because past ideas or recollections would be related to one another or to the patient's present thoughts. In this new kind of association the fragments of content tended, according to him, to 'hover side by side' in an all-pervasive 'excess of discernment'. A simple example of this 'hovering' of delusional contents might be:

> As a child I once fell into the water. My sister was standing there. That is it.

This peculiar form of association makes it possible to understand how a delusional interpretation can exist side by side with an everyday interpretation of reality. It also explains the difficulty in defining:

> the borderlines between sudden ideas, ill-defined delusional associations, frank delusions and simple casual interpretations.

He stressed that there was a 'flux and reflux of ingredients' which operated against the persistence of delusion. Whether process-like primary ideas should be described as delusional or not depends on their duration and on the role of the primary delusional idea as initiator of further thought processes with a similar direction. Primary delusional thought processes should, he believed, be regarded as a definite delusion only if they are held with conviction, whether based on recent experience or rooted in the qualities and strivings of the personality.

Carl Schneider did not know where in the 'flux and reflux of ingredients' a delusion begins or ends. He regarded it merely as a by-product of the underlying formal thought disorder. Zucker came to a similar conclusion from experiments on imagery involving schizophrenics with good powers of self-description. Zucker claimed that the experience of significance is always associated with changes in the primary content of the image. Thus a patient was asked to imagine a dog in a garden, jumping over a wall, and running after a milk float. The patient reported the relationship:

> Dog runs after cart – driver stops hitting the horse – all cruelty to animals will cease.

From numerous examples of this kind, some of them not quite so convincing as the one quoted, Zucker demonstrated the connection between the experience of significance and the secondary change in the process of imagination. So far as the spontaneous schizophrenic experience is concerned, however, he found himself confronted with the difficulty that he could not demonstrate any secondary image which was related in content to the creation of significance. How Zucker attempted to overcome this difficulty can be read in his highly original and stimulating work on the *Functional Analysis of Schizophrenia* (1939). The sense of significance, he claimed, could only develop if images were induced in rapid succession and if the capacity for self-observation were still intact. If the latter were lost completely, incoherence and talking past the point began to appear. Zucker mentioned two situations in which such experiences of significance could lead to a florid psychosis – if a subject with premorbid paranoid traits entered a mood of grandiose expectations, or if another person, not necessarily paranoid by nature, were driven into a state of perplexity with loss of meaningful orientations.

Neither Carl Schneider nor Zucker had much use for Jaspers' differentiation between delusional perceptions, ideas and awareness. Both these writers believed that it was of little consequence for the actual functioning of the delusional process whether it took the form of a perception or an idea.

Berze & Gruhle (1929) did not apply Carl Schneider's concept of thought fusion to hazy relationships between heterogenous contents, but reserved it rather for cases in which two thoughts, perceptions, desires or affects merged, as it were, into a primary unit. In Gruhle's example of the schizophrenic who saw three marble-topped tables and knew at once that the end of the world was at hand, the idea of the end of the world merged with the incidental perception of the tables to form an integral whole. In this way the character of immediate revelation, which is traditionally specific only for perceptions, is extended to the unit created by this fusion, so that the notion of the end of the world equally acquires the quality of immediate certainty. The certainty attached to the idea came at a stroke together with the perception. Berze saw in this fusion of thoughts coupled with subsequent explanations a basic principle that applied in many cases of schizophrenic association. He claimed that the lack of logical relationship is only an apparent one, as the patient's thinking acquires an underlying quality of consistency because of persistent attitudes, persistent isolated notions or mood states.

Kronfeld (1930) took Carl Schneider's notions a step further and asked what was behind these formal characteristics of schizophrenic thinking. In fact, he claimed that it was not the formal rules of thinking that were primarily altered, but the material available to them, by which Kronfeld meant original, dark and unusual experiential constellations or 'mood states'. To come to terms with them, he claimed, called for particular modes of mental activity which do not exist, and hence the formal thought disorder, which Carl Schneider talked about, emerged secondarily as an attempt to rationalise them. These mood states appeared as delusional feelings, such as suspiciousness and altered significance of the self. Vague experiences of reference developed, which were transferred to the external world, threatening the patient's self or 'self-ness'. This projection was supported by certain sensory components of the mood state, which encouraged the subject to believe that something significant was happening to him externally. Kronfeld believed that there was a psychological continuum – from the 'organismic mood state' via the delusional mood state and delusion-like feelings to sensory misperceptions (i.e. delusional perceptions), delusional judgements and delusional awareness. This formulation does not contribute any substantially new insights into the nature of the delusional mood state. Further, constructs such as 'sensory components' seem to me too artificial, and the concept of 'delusional-like feelings' is too ill-defined. Nevertheless, Kronfeld deserves credit for having drawn our attention to certain important psychological facts inherent in the delusional experience.

Ontological approach (delusion as an attempt on the part of a subject to give meaning to his new existence)

Storch (1922), in what he calls an 'existential-analytical exercise', criticises phenomenologists such as Gruhle for merely providing formal definitions 'well outside a genuine understanding of schizophrenia'. Storch's portrayal of the world of incipient schizophrenia as 'peculiarly insubstantial, evanescent and hovering' reminds us superficially of the formulations of Carl Schneider, but he places more emphasis on what he calls the 'archaic and primitive' nature of the thought disorder. He considers that in this way the schizophrenic 'becomes transparent to himself and reaches through to himself'. Kunz (1931) considers that the essential happening, that which is primary and fundamental in a schizophrenic delusion, is not the delusional quality, but rather the whole alteration of existence, the total change in 'being in the world'. Just as the delusions of the melancholic represent his effort to explain his depression, so the schizophrenic primary delusion is a reflection of the change of existence – with the difference that the primary delusion is the only way in which the subject's change of existence can be experienced and expressed.

Kurt Schneider found it difficult to understand why this change of existence should be expressed in the form of a delusion, although this might be an acceptable explanation in the relatively few patients who display delusional mood states. Paranoid delusions in schizophrenics, for example, can easily be explained as disorders of thinking and judgement. Von Baeyer (1932), however, pointed out that the two approaches, functional and ontological, are required to give a comprehensive account of the form and content of a delusion. On the one hand, a purely functional explanation of delusions is not enough, as it fails to explain why this function change does not cover individually random contents, but is confined to quite definite themes such as persecution, jealousy, catastrophe and redemption. On the other hand, it is not possible to interpret the functional features satisfactorily in terms of a global existential change.

Causes of primary delusion
The cause of a primary delusion is not a subject that comes within the scope of the descriptive approach. Generally, the writers we have been discussing are content with a reference to some hypothetical disease process or else they assume a personality change. The delusional mood state is the primary pathological experience, which Jaspers regarded as the source but not the motive of a primary delusion. A reference to premorbid personality might explain the content, the theme of the delusion, but never the delusion itself, that is to say the actual existence of a delusion. Carl Schneider's solution, to regard the cause of delusion as an abnormality in the formal mode of thinking of the patient, is an exception, but he still leaves unexplained the cause of this formal thought disorder. Berze had originally put forward a theory which explained delusions of reference in terms of disturbances of perception. He considered at that time that there was a 'pathological tone which, so to speak, passes from the act of perception to the object perceived'. He later modified his theory by introducing a new characteristic, namely a factor of uncertainty in the grasp of the object, this being derived from a disturbance of apperception. Since these uncertainties were transferred on to the object in the same way as the disagreeable feelings, the object perceived would seem to the patient changed, puzzling and suspicious. In these 'feelings', however, it was the intellectual rather than the emotional content which was important. Yet later he modified

the theory again, proposing that the primary element is a change in the process of perception occurring as part of the phenomena produced by a general insufficiency of activity. Berze's final views were mentioned in connection with Carl Schneider's concept of thought fusion.

It should be noted with all these theories of the cause of primary delusion that, if it were possible to derive a primary delusion from one of the closely related primary symptoms with which it is intimately associated, or from some underlying disorder, then it would no longer be a primary but a secondary delusion, and there would be no such thing as a genuine delusion.

Part 1b – Descriptive studies of secondary delusion

Delusion-like ideas, in contrast to genuine delusional ideas, can be derived from motives. We can also include sudden delusional notions here, in so far as they answer the criterion of understandability or 'explicability in terms of motives' as proposed by Kurt Schneider.

The delusional ideas found in manic-depressive illness are, according to Gruhle and others, verbal representations of the expansive or depressive background state. The depressed patient's delusions of insignificance, nothingness, guilt, metamorphosis and demonic possession, like his hypochondriacal attitudes, largely reflect his self-denial, self-abasement or anxiety. The patient who wants to denigrate and torture himself speaks of the grave of his children being dug in the room next door, feels that people avoid him, look at him askance and abandon him. This type of persecutory delusion, however, represents only a tendency for self-destruction. Manic delusional ideas, on the other hand, are more in the nature of showing off, or reflect feelings of happiness and self aggrandisement, and take the form of shifting, playful ideas. They resemble the delusions found in general paralysis, which, no matter what their content, have always a grandiose orientation. Nearly everything that comes to mind in the form of perception, image or idea, has the hallmark of grandeur. There can be no doubt that these sudden delusional ideas, especially when they occur in cyclothymic, manic or depressed patients, are inspired by the background mood. Whether the extreme degree of exaggeration frequently attached to them can also be directly derived from the mood depends on the extent to which one accepts the criterion of empathy and understanding. Hoche (1934) would deny that melancholic delusional ideas represent attempts to rationalise anxiety, but sees them rather as equally valid symptoms and co-ordinates of the abnormal mood.

The next group of secondary delusional ideas which we should mention are based largely on hallucinations. They are often interpreted as a kind of 'explanatory delusion' (Wernicke) in the sense of the 'inborn law of causality' (Griesinger). Patients who hear voices, or experience abnormal bodily sensations and similar phenomena, conclude that these things must be caused by external influences such as radio, thought transference, hypnosis or magic. The further elaboration of such thoughts to form a fixed system of secondary delusions of persecution generally occurs only when the morbid process persists and with it the hallucinations or other abnormal experiences which have caused the delusions. It is of course not a matter of logical deduction such as might be made by a normal person in similar circumstances. If, for example, a patient who has just recovered from a toxic confusional state clings briefly to his hallucinations, this should hardly, according to Kurt Schneider, be regarded as a delusion. Wyrsch (1935) would in such cases speak of a simple belief in the reality of these sensory deceptions. Although the dependence of delusions on hallucinations may be regarded by some as an antiquated idea, it is undoubtedly a matter of observed fact. Nor can it be overruled by Aschaffenburg's objection that it is the content of thought which determines the content of hallucinations, rather than the existence of a sensory illusion, unconnected with the patient's ego and alien to it, which lends delusional direction to his thoughts. Both can undoubtedly occur.

A delusion can furthermore be derived from other schizophrenic phenomena, particularly thought insertion. A primary delusion may be further elaborated in the context of the rest of the patient's mental life, giving rise to a new delusion. 'Old' delusions may undergo secondary change as their hold on a subject wanes.

In organic psychoses, the 'exogenous reactions' of Bonhoeffer, delusions are usually explicable in terms of hallucinations or disturbances of judgement associated with clouding of consciousness.

In psychopathic personalities, delusional formation is derived from emotions and is amenable to empathy. These are discussed in more detail below. Gruhle regards it as incorrect to extend the concept of delusion to the symptoms of psychopathic personalities who habitually incline to the view that they are being slighted and not properly appreciated. Hedenberg called these 'synthetic-affective delusional ideas'. They are usually personal creations, in keeping with normal life, but where judgement is based on an existing personal system of opinions, bearing traces of the influence of an affective motive. Transitions between such psychopathic 'delusions', if they deserve this label, and the typical schizophrenic delusion are emphatically denied by almost all the authors quoted so far.

Part 2 – Explanation of the origin of delusion

A – *Definition of delusion*

Before discussing the understandable and causal relationships of a delusion, I shall present a brief review of the definitions of delusion commonly used in this field.

The definition given in the ninth edition of Kraepelin's textbook, partially revised by Lange (1927), that:

> delusional ideas are pathologically derived errors, not amenable to correction by logical proof to the contrary

is basically on the same lines as Kraepelin's formulation of 1883, that:

> Every delusional idea is a pathologically distorted notion.

At that time, however, it was superstition rather than error which was postulated as the psychological flaw. Bumke's formulation (1936) of a delusional idea as a 'pathologically generated and at the same time incorrigible error' was no real advance on Ziehen's view, that it was a form of pathological error, or Hoche's, that it was a 'pathologically distorted and incorrigible notion', both suggested before the period covered by this article.

Someone who persistently adheres to a demonstrably incorrect and nonsensical idea is, of course, not necessarily labouring under a delusion:

> There is no delusional idea held by the mentally ill which cannot be exceeded in its absurdity by the convictions of fanatics, either as individuals or en masse. (Hoche 1934)

At the same time a delusion is by no means always incorrigible, nor indeed incorrect in content – delusional relationships may accidentally coincide with a real state of affairs. Objective inaccuracy, at least in the case of delusions which come within the bounds of possibility, is certainly no criterion. Nor does the egocentricity of a delusion, which in any case is not always present, distinguish it from belief. The fact that a delusion is primarily an individual phenomenon does not help us to decide whether someone is a prophet or a madman. According to Hoppe (1919), who has written the most informed work on the relationship between delusion and belief, the only criterion is the cultural value of the idea in question. Even so, it is possible for a mentally ill person to have certain ideas with a cultural value. Nor does it seem to be a very happy solution to distinguish delusions from overvalued ideas by following Jossmann's suggestion (1921) that a delusion is a misinterpretation, while an overvalued idea is an error. According to Birnbaum (1915), the overvalued idea can be a prodromal stage of a delusion, particularly in psychopathic cases. In summary, no one has yet discovered a way of defining a delusion without invoking the aid of an underlying pathological process. Yet, according to Aschaffenburg's critique of 1915, the word 'pathological' pre-empts the very search for those criteria which make it pathological.

Bleuler (1937) and Jahrreiss (1928) already include a causal notion in their definitions.

> Delusional ideas are incorrect notions which have arisen not from an incidental failure of logic, but rather from an inner need. (Bleuler)

> The delusional idea is an error created by a morbidly altered feeling of significance; it is not amenable to correction, as it is experienced with unshakable certainty. In psychodynamic terms it is possible to arrange delusional ideas in a sequence that ranges from strong affective tensions giving rise to slight changes in feelings of significance at one extreme, to delusional ideas arising from a primary change in feelings of significance and with affective factors playing only a secondary role at the other. (Jahrreiss)

Most phenomenologists reject this attempt to bridge the gap between a 'delusion' and delusion-like ideas. They see a fundamental and unbridgeable difference between the sense of being noticed, such as a young soldier might experience on appearing in uniform for the first time in public, and the inexplicable delusions of reference of the schizophrenic. Others, however, disagree. Lange (1927) refuses to concede Jaspers' differentiation between genuine delusions and delusion-like ideas. In his view, the schizophrenic experiences of significance are closely related to hallucinations. And Bumke (1936) cannot see any sense in defining a 'delusion' in such a way that it can only be found, with rare exceptions, in cases of schizophrenia.

B – Understandable explanations of delusion

Personality disorder

Gaupp had been one of the earliest psychiatrists to draw attention to the close relationship between personality and psychosis, pointing to certain forms of paranoid disposition and 'abortive paranoia'. He elaborated the thesis from 1914 onwards in numerous papers based on the case of the headmaster Wagner. The necessary basis of Wagner's paranoia, according to Gaupp, was a combination of anxious paranoid and sensitive personality traits, overvalued feelings of sexual guilt, and a sense of suspicion and exaggerated self-esteem. In contrast to Kraepelin's view that paranoia has an insidious onset, Wagner's illness started abruptly as an acute reaction to a homosexual incident. He interpreted the delusional self-reference as a projection of a mood of anxious self-torture, a process which Wagner himself described in the following way:

> I would interpret certain things which had been said to me as if they had actually happened to me. I suppose many were only irrelevant happenings and coincidences but to me they appeared intentional. Of course I need not have interpreted them in this way, but the things which fill one's mind, one is only too ready to place into the minds of others.

The main theme of Wagner's self-reference was sexual guilt, a constant feature for many years, and Gaupp placed particular emphasis on this in distinguishing Wagner's experiences from those seen in more diffuse states with delusions of reference. Another unusual feature which Gaupp emphasised was the fluctuation of the delusional ideas with changes in the patient's life situation. The ideas of self-reference would flare up whenever external events gave cause for concern. These observations were not in keeping with Kraepelin's view of paranoia as an unshakable delusional system brought about by inner causes and of insidious development. The second part of Kraepelin's definition of paranoia, the preservation of complete clarity and orderliness of thought, volition and behaviour, did however apply unequivocally to Wagner' case throughout decades of observation and right up to the time of his death.

The case of Wagner, and Gaupp's interpretation of it, provoked controversy amongst psychiatrists. Lange, for example, commented that:

> Everyone who has concerned himself with Wagner has interpreted him in a different way.

Gaupp's view was that his particular personality made him vulnerable both to unusual life events and his own biological milestones with the result that eventually a paranoid and alien transformation into psychosis took place. The separation of 'development' and 'process', stressed by most psychiatrists, was less important in Gaupp's formulation. Another issue which emerges from Wagner's biography is the relationship between delusions of persecution and delusions of grandeur, about which Wagner himself spoke. The relationship in this case appears to confirm the traditional view that delusions of grandeur are secondary, although it is not the degree of persecution itself but the degree of suffering as a result of the persecution that inspires the ideas of grandeur. Wagner, however, had always shown a tendency to self-aggrandisement – his confessions are especially convincing in this respect – and, for this reason, we cannot be sure that his case confirms the traditional view on the relationship between these two types of delusion.

Kretschmer's approach to the relationship between personality and delusional illness is marked by a thoroughness unsurpassed by any other writer. He distinguishes three personality types which are prone to delusional development: the quarrelsome paranoiac; the sensitive, conscience-driven paranoiac; and the wishful paranoiac.

In the sensitive character there is conflict between softness and vulnerability and an ambitious element. The key experience of the sensitive paranoiac is the experience of shameful inadequacy, of failure in the sexual or moral sphere of life. This experience is then suppressed and assumes the form of a 'complex'. If pressure from within is sufficiently intense, this will result in the projection of affect, that is to say the sense of shame is reflected and transformed into a perceptible symbol, namely the observation that the environment knows about and despises the patient's inner world. In its milder form this sense of reference need not be seen as outside the range of normal, but it can progress to become a firmly held delusion of reference. A sensitive delusion of reference is thus an enlarged mirror image of the sensitive personality. For it to be pathological, according to Kretschmer, the self-reference must be 'systematic, massive and minutely detailed'. On the one hand, it can be distinguished from an ordinary paranoid response which might result from feeling slighted or injured in some way. On the other hand it differs from the delusions of reference which occur in schizophrenia or paraphrenia for which one can have no empathy and which run a course independently of actual experience. Kretschmer distinguished three varieties according to the course of the illness: 'psychopathic reaction', in which there was complete remission; a 'permanent reference neurosis', in which the natural disposition, once disturbed, could not find its way back to its original state; and a 'habitual reference neurosis' which evolved without any special precipitating experiences other than those that accompany the different ages of man.

The second main group – the quarrelsome or querulant paranoiac – developed, according to Kretschmer, from a personality in which two opposing traits co-existed – marked mental energy coupled with latent feelings of inadequacy. The actual delusion could be one of jealousy or persecution, and the general clinical picture resembled that seen in sensitive delusions of reference, except that a sense of personal guilt was usually lacking.

The third group is that of the wish psychosis, the psychosis of the naively euphoric dreamer. Conflict is not essential, as in the other two groups, and the usual manifestation is a chronic delusion of being loved, which differs only quantitatively from the mental set of normal people in love.

All three types of paranoia require a particular form of inner experience and not the raw material of a life event for their development. The callous infringement of legal rights which the psychopath sees in a hole in the fence, the sin seen in unrevealed love, and the call of God read into a passage in the Bible are all inner experiences from which the paranoid state derives. In view of the large number of types Kretschmer concluded that 'there are paranoid people, but no such thing as paranoia'. Delusional development primarily based on personality factors is further reinforced by life events, milieu, such physical factors as weakness of the sexual constitution, endogenous loading, and a variety of debilitating conditions such as head injury, exhaustion and involution. With the help of a multidimensional diagnostic approach it would be possible to interpret the interweavings of endogenous and reactive components and even to understand early cases of schizophrenia and paraphrenia precipitated by life events.

Kurt Schneider was rather critical of the concept of sensitive delusions of reference. He based his comments on the case of Katarina Schroth, who, like Kretschmer's Helene Renner and Anna Feldweg, was of lower middle class background and sensitive disposition, and manifested a similar psychosis, but in whom the precipitating experience of shameful failure, namely that of a secret and hopeless love, was lacking. In her case the first encounter with the loved one was undoubtedly a primary delusional experience itself, and Schneider suggested that the love experiences in Kretschmer's cases were in fact delusional from the outset and not a reaction at all. Since a number of psychotic states derive their content from similar experience, for example shame at masturbation, it seemed to Schneider that a 'reactive' component was not specific to sensitive delusions of reference, a criticism which largely undermined their distinct nosological status. Kehrer attacked the other *sine qua non*, the issue of a sensitive personality. From his observations in the case of Else Boss he found that typical delusions of reference with a sexual or moral theme could also occur in people who are not of sensitive character at all. Lange cast further doubt on the concept by describing sensitive people who demonstrably had had morally shaming experiences but in whom, contrary to expectations, sensitive delusions of reference failed to develop, and insecure but not sensible people who underwent reversible paranoid illnesses. Finally, Langelueddeke (1926) presented the case of a patient with sensitive paranoia, the psychotic contents of which were initially understandable but with a subsequent course that was unequivocally consistent with a schizophrenic illness.

Inner conflicts and emotions

According to Bleuler (1926), the formation of delusions depends on the balance between emotional attachment to something and the firmness of logical associations. The logical processes may be too weak, as in schizophrenic thought disorder, or emotional attachment too strong, as in paranoia. Emotionally-laden complexes representing some chronic conflict between wish and reality, and repressed complexes representing an individual's own inferiority, may become so powerful that they cause delusional ideas – delusions of persecution, in which failure is blamed on others, or delusions of grandeur, in which wishes become fulfilled facts.

Kehrer (1922) also placed more emphasis on specific inner conflicts than on whether a subject fitted broad personality types. In particular, it was the social component to his life, and the conflict between sexual and social drives, which he thought critical for delusional formation. For one person the greatest ideal in life might be his moral standing, for another his honour, and for a third his sexual potency. If he then finds himself far removed from realising this aspiration, and suffers in secret the shipwreck of all that forms the goal of his most noble ambitions, this, according to Kehrer, is the fundamental condition for the development of paranoia. It may begin with what he calls a subclinical paranoid attitude, a mild tendency to delusional interpretation of life events. At this stage the different misinterpretations are only loosely linked, like pieces on a chess board, and a fixed delusion is avoided. Later, when unusual events are encountered, true delusional interpretation ensues.

Schulte (1924) tried to resolve the problem of paranoia in terms of a disordered sense of belonging. According to him, there are people who are unable to achieve a sense of belonging to some group, either for external reasons, such as language barrier, deafness or imprisonment, or internal reasons – they cannot 'play the game any longer'. They resolve their conflict by restructuring their relationship with the group: instead of feeling hurt or envious about their exclusion, they reinterpret their situation in a persecutory sense. If they cannot achieve a sense of true togetherness, they make do with a substitute, the togetherness of the persecutor and persecuted. As Gruhle put it:

> To be lonely is impossible, but to be persecuted, that is possible.

There is something appealing in these ideas of Schulte, which reminds one of Freud's remarks on the origin of paranoid delusions in the case of Daniel Schreber. Schulte's account is echoed by other writers, for example Kahn (1929):

> Far better to fight the whole world, or to suffer under the whole world, than to be lonely.

All delusions, to some extent, isolate the individual from the outside world. Each event they encounter forces the question: 'What meaning does this have for me in my loneliness?' When the accumulated tension involved in the escape from loneliness, in certain individuals, reaches a certain level, a delusion emerges, supplying, as it were, the missing pieces in the world puzzle. In this sense, a delusion has a meaning and a purpose – the preservation and rescue of self-values, leading to a heightening of self-esteem.

Otto Kant (1927) claimed to have found a measure of what a delusion represents by studying the extent to which it corresponded with reality. He observed that the behaviour of the deluded patient with respect to reality (i.e. did they act on their beliefs) generally lagged behind their subjective notion of reality (i.e. the conviction with which the belief was held). This is a common observation in psychotic individuals, that despite their apparent absolute conviction in something, they rarely act as if it were true. Kant took this to mean that a delusion functioned as a kind of valve, enabling a deluded subject to abreact his hate and guilt onto the outside world. Of course, in some deluded individuals, action and certainty of belief have the same 'reality weighting' with dramatic results, such as murder. But Kant believed that such exact correspondence was rare. Kant's views on the thwarting of inner needs by social forces are similar to Adler's, but he goes further and incorporates Freud's notion of 'wish reversal', which in the case of paranoia means the conversion of a need for a relationship into a sense of persecution. He attempts to explain away the paradox, inexplicable at first sight even to him, that delusions of persecution should contain a wish, by reference to everyday self-deceptions, and by invoking Nietzsche's comment that a self-deception involves a discrepancy between a subjective experience and the motivating forces behind it. Finally he claims to find understandable even schizophrenic delusions, which virtually all writers on psychopathology agree is impossible. He claims that their understandability can be uncovered at the deepest layer of mental life, inaccessible to consciousness, and where, he assumes, a perceived threat to vital functions is taking place. This threat is dealt with by autistic detachment from reality, emotional change and the use of archaic modes of thinking. It must be said that his explanation is a thoroughly tangled interplay of factors, adduced from a variety of sources.

Psychodynamic approaches to delusion usually borrow freely from the chief exponents of 'depth psychology' – Freud, Adler and Jung. Their writings on delusion are characterised by an emphasis on the purpose and meaning of a delusion for the individual. Even Kraepelin wrote about 'the need to form delusions' and Bleuler, as is well known, was strongly influenced by Freud and Jung. Most approaches of this nature are specious and teleological, as they treat 'cause' and 'purpose' as if they were synonymous. Despite this obvious fallacy, many authors who do not primarily subscribe to a dynamic position have felt obliged to adopt a teleological position. Kronfeld, for example, saw in some types of delusional content a grandiose attempt by the individual to regain his identity, and Kunz regarded primary delusion as a schizophrenic change of existence. Mayer-Gross (1932), not known for his psychodynamic orientation, also recognised meaningful tendencies in the delusional experience: an attempt on the part of the patient to render meaningful the situation in which he found himself. Even Jaspers left open the question of the extent to which the contents of a primary delusion had symbolic significance. Ewald (1919) suggested a compromise, whereby a delusion as such emanated from an abnormal personality structure, but its form was the consequence of the personality damage inflicted by the schizophrenic illness. Undoubtedly the content, even of a primary delusion, can be explored from many different points of view, and the psychodynamic approach is appealing, only because the strict phenomenological approach has been essentially sterile.

External conflict

There is a consensus of opinion regarding the nature of delusions which are psychogenic or reactive in kind. They include delusions of persecution encountered among the *deaf*, the *blind* and those isolated by a *language barrier*. *Mentally subnormal* soldiers, after transfer to another regiment, developed a paranoid delusional state, according to Herschmann (1919), and Kurt Schneider showed how delusions of reference could develop after a violent attack of fear. Hesse (1936) described paranoid states in febrile delirium, in which clouding of consciousness creates the right conditions for the appearance of delusional ideas. The same principle applies to delusional states caused by cerebral trauma. In all these physical conditions, however, one presupposes the existence of an abnormal premorbid personality which facilitates the delusional formations.

Several authors have analysed the factors which give rise to psychoses in prisoners. According to Foersterling (1923), the basic element of a genuine paranoid prison reaction was:

> a demonstrable need for a delusion . . . to fill all that emptiness with something positive . . . to install sense, meaning and purpose to their situation . . . and to allow a flight from reality.

Other authors have emphasised the simulation which such psychoses represented, and Knigge (1935) the hysterical component.

Other life experiences and situations have been compared with those of a prisoner, and the same factors – wish fulfilment, flight from reality – have been invoked in these cases. Delusional states specific to governesses, primary school teachers and dissatisfied school masters have all been described, although the subject is no longer topical. Litiginous individuals seeking accident compensation are, however, considered by many authorities, including Kraepelin, vulnerable to delusional formation. There is dispute, however, about the nature of the delusional state. Some authors regard it as typical paranoia. Kraepelin, for example, considered that there was always some kind of defeat which had precipitated the condition and, if this were true, litiginous paranoia would indeed be a typical example of a delusion brought about by external conflict. Wetzel (1922) questioned this formulation with a detailed account of the case of Freiherr von Hausen, an extraordinarily litigious individual. According to Wetzel:

> In von Hausen's case there was never any central reference point for his delusions, no concentric waves of paranoia emanating from such a point. Instead, there were countless intersecting circles, the centres of which would provide, at any one moment, the point at which he would once again come into conflict with the law. Von Hausen, despite his obstinacy, was by no means impervious to reason, and had in fact frequently suffered injustice.

The case of von Hausen, as presented by Wetzel, undermined the classic concept of litigious paranoia, as one finds it described in earlier textbooks. It encouraged Kolle, for example, to object to the use of the term delusional state at all in this context. He preferred the term 'justice neurosis'.

So-called 'induced madness' – *folie à deux* – also belongs to Kraepelin's exogenous paranoid disorders. In such cases the external factor is the inducer, the 'delusional transmitter'. However, it is usually incorrect to regard the condition as 'induced madness' because one is not dealing with a mental illness, but merely an abnormal reaction with borrowed content. For this reason there have been few papers on the subject over the period reviewed in this article. Most authorities now accept, as they accept the demise of the concept of litigious paranoia, that the main variety of *folie à deux, folie imposée*, is not a true delusional state but a temporary acceptance of certain beliefs by suggestible individuals. Some authors refer to this as an 'apparent psychosis'. The other two varieties have greater claim to be regarded as delusional states, but are rare. *Folie transformée*, in which delusions from one individual's psychosis are transferred and incorporated into a pre-existing psychosis in another individual, is one variety. *Folie communiquée*, in which a previously sane individual takes over and elaborates the abnormal beliefs of another, is particularly rare.

One relatively undisputed area is the importance of mental subnormality in generating delusional states. Neustadt (1928) claimed that mentally subnormal individuals had an emotional life which made them particularly liable to suspiciousness. He believed, however, that they would never develop a systematised paranoia because they lacked the capacity to elaborate ideas according to broad principles.

C – Causal explanations of delusion
Constitution
[This section deals with constitutional determinants of personality – e.g. psychophysiological reactivity, mental set – as opposed to acquired influences on personality encountered during life which was the subject of the section on personality disorder in Part 2B. There is some overlap, and the division between constitution and acquired personality disorder reflects the different orientations of biological and psychodynamic psychiatrists rather than any true division of personality itself, Tr.]

Kraepelin believed that paranoia developed in those individuals who were constitutionally abnormal, in that their reaction to life events was different in some way, and their reasoning processes impaired, the latter due to retarded development. He considered that a life-long heightening of self-consciousness could lead to delusions of grandeur, and a hypersensitivity to the environment to delusions of persecution. He admitted that some individuals could become deluded as a consequence of understandable facets of their personality (as in Kretschmer's cases and the other ways discussed in section 2B); in other individuals delusions were generated by an abnormality in the constitutional factors affecting personality; in yet other individuals there might be abnormalities in both sets of personality determinant.

Lange, however, whose point of view is similar to that of his teacher Kraepelin, could not identify any definite constitutional factor which distinguished paranoid subjects from the rest of the population. He mentions only the most nonspecific personality traits, such as emotional reactivity, egoism, a non-schizophrenic 'woolliness of thinking' and certain mannerisms. To explain the excessive self-centredness of the paranoid individual he introduces the concept of mental rigidity, but how this itself comes about is left unexplained. In the end his explanation for the existence of paranoid individuals is trivial and virtually tautologous: paranoid subjects are those who possess to an exaggerated degree a normally occurring and widely distributed trait.

Manic-depressive illness

Specht had taught that, if one regarded suspiciousness as an affect, then paranoia became a major affective psychosis equal in status to mania and depressive psychosis. Other writers followed this approach, noting that anger, indignation and rage were also types of affect which were common to all three psychoses. Stoecker (1919) maintained that all delusional contents could be reduced to four basic affects – depression, elation, anxiety and suspiciousness – and that paranoia was fundamentally an affective disorder coloured by a premorbid paranoid disposition. Ewald (1919) claimed that it was often difficult to distinguish whether delusions of persecution were a psychopathic manifestation or a variant of manic-depressive illness. The critical factor appeared to be whether the subject had a personality which made him self-centred – which favoured the development of paranoia – or was orientated towards life and living – which favoured manic-depressive illness. Other writers, for example Kolle, are prepared to accept that a cyclothymic personality contributes to the development of a paranoid psychosis. It should be noted, however, that the word 'affect' is used rather broadly in some formulations. Fankhauser (1931), for example, considers paranoia to be the third affective psychosis alongside mania and melancholia, not because of a cyclothymic element in the premorbid personality, but because of a 'morbid ideational affect'. What he means by this is similar to what Bleuler (see page 124) meant by undue emotional adherence to an idea. A powerful emotional attachment to something, however, cannot be simply equated with the existence of an affective psychosis.

Cerebral dysfunction

There are numerous attempts in the literature to explain delusional formation by specific kinds of cerebral dysfunction. At the beginning of the period covered by this article it was fashionable to adopt the principles of association psychology. Such notions as a deterioration of the connections between a 'self sphere' and a 'world sphere' and dissociation of certain 'idea centres' from the rest of the cortex were entertained. Others proposed excessive irritability or hyperaesthesia of specific cerebral regions. Iwanow-Smolensky (1926), a disciple of Pavlov, suggested an endogenous irritability of the 'centre for the unconditioned reflex of self-defence'.

In general, however, most authors have rejected any primary contribution of cerebral damage, even in the genesis of delusions of jealousy in alcoholics, where toxic effects on the brain, although certainly present, are regarded as incidental.

Sexuality

There is no need to enumerate the varied mechanisms whereby sexuality has been held responsible for the genesis of a delusion. Thorough and scientifically valid studies on the matter, however, do not exist and the most one can say is that sexuality is important in shaping a psychosis in Birnbaum's pathoplastic sense. Mayer-Gross also noted that sexual deviation is more likely to be a consequence than a cause of a delusional state, a salutary reminder that all putative explanations of delusion may well be effect rather than cause.

Life epoch

Age has been implicated as a cause of delusional states because of the difference between psychoses of middle age and those of the elderly. One might expect the old to blame others for what they regard as their failure to accomplish certain goals. This has been put forward as an explanation for sensitive delusions of reference in ageing spinsters and for delusions of jealousy in men in the climacteric. Organic psychiatrists, such as Kleist, had suggested, before the period reviewed in this article, that a subclinical paranoid disposition could be converted into a florid paranoid psychosis in the involutional period by hormonal changes which were occurring at this time. Other writers dispute this organic explanation, and some, for example Mosbacher (1931), doubt whether there is such a thing as an endogenous delusional illness specific to later epochs of life.

The majority of authors, who deny a pathogenic effect of increasing age, readily admit that it colours the content of a delusion. Such themes as sex, fear of personal injury and prejudice are common. These themes, particularly that of prejudice, reflect the thoughts and feelings at that age. Further characteristics of small-mindedness and poverty of interests can also be recognised. Even delusions of grandeur in the elderly sometimes have a quality of stinginess about them. Kraepelin pointed out that delusions of poverty, nihilistic delusions and hypochondriacal delusions never occur in the young. He also believed that paranoia, as a classical illness of middle life, represents the tendency in maturer years to take issue with the world and to form independent views of life and the world. Kraepelin explains the rarity of delusional ideas in youth and childhood in terms of a more fleeting and emotional elaboration of the environment, which was a less favourable substrate for the development of delusions. Homburger (1926) observes that children, by virtue of their suggestibility, superficiality and easily deflected attention, lack the kind of perseverance and capacity for prolonged ruminations on ideas in all their ramifications which are necessary for the formation of systematised delusions. The gloomy, painful and enquiring condition of a delusional mood is quite alien to children.

Regression to an earlier stage of development
Several writers have tried to explain schizophrenic delusions and thinking by comparing them with the way children or primitive people are assumed to think and believe. Reiss (1921) suggested that such primitive modes of thinking might be revived, if there were a relaxation of the inhibition exerted on them by the more recently acquired logical thinking. Schilder was also committed to this view, in which, as he saw it, schizophrenic and primitive views of the world shared a similar psychological projection of the individual, with the result that the individual came to believe that he controlled outside events. Storch tried to identify common qualities in the thinking of schizophrenics and primitive people, for example a tendency to condense heterogenous elements of things into a single meaningful entity, and 'displacement', a tendency to select one small feature of a thing as a representation of the whole. A general tendency to make concrete analogies from

abstract concepts is often mentioned in comparative discussions of this kind but, as several writers have pointed out, similarities between the two states of mind may be incidental, and there is no strong reason to suppose a causal link. Von Baeyer was heavily critical of all such developmental hypotheses. In the first place, he commented, the development of an individual through various stages has nothing intrinsically to do with the development of mankind and its culture. Secondly, he denied the fact that primitive thought processes were characteristic of schizophrenia, especially the hebephrenic subtype. And thirdly, he pointed out the clear difference between the autochthonous psychotic experience of a schizophrenic and the understandable superstitions of a healthy individual.

References

Aschaffenburg, G. (1915) Allgemeine Symptomatologie der Psychosen. In *Handbuch der Psychiatrie*, ed. G. Aschaffenburg. Leipzig & Wein: F. Deuticke.

Berze, J. & Gruhle, H. W. (1929) *Psychologie der Schizophrenie*. Berlin: Springer.

Birnbaum, K. (1915) Zur Paranoiafrage. *Zeitschrift für die gesamte Neurologie und Psychiatrie* **29**, 305–22.

Bleuler, E. (1926) *Affektivität, Suggestibilität, Paranoia*, 2nd edn. Halle: Harhold.

Bleuler, E. (1937) *Lehrbuch der Psychiatrie*, 6th edn. Berlin: Springer.

Bumke, O. (1936) *Lehrbuch der Geisteskrankheiten*, 4th edn. München: J. F. Bergmann.

Ewald, G. (1919) Paranoia und manisch-depressives Irresein. *Zeitschrift für die gesamte Neurologie und Psychiatrie* **49**, 270–326.

Fankhauser, E. (1931) Gefühl, Affekt und Stimmung: manisch-depressives Irresein, Paranoia. *Zeitschrift für die gesamte Neurologie und Psychiatrie* **132**, 333–66.

Foersterling, W. (1923) Paranoia bei Kriminale. *Monatsschrift für Psychiatrie und Neurologie* **19**, 1–27.

Gaupp, R. & Wollenberg, R. (1914) *Zur Psychologie des Massenmords Hauptlehrer Wagner von Degerloch*. Berlin: Springer.

Gruhle, H. W. (1915) Selbstschilderung und Einfühlung. *Zeitschrift für die gesamte Neurologie und Psychiatrie* **28**, 148–231.

Hedenberg, S. (1927) Über die synthetisch-affektiven und schizophrenen Wahnideen. *Archiv für Psychiatrie und Nervenkrankheiten* **80**, 665–751.

Herschmann, H. (1921) Bemerkungen zu der Arbeit von Rudolf Allers. *Zeitschrift für die gesamte Neurologie und Psychiatrie* **66**, 346.

Hesse, H. (1936) Über Hintergrundreaktionen. *Nervenarzt* **9**, 227–33.

Heveroch, A. (1919) Der Beziehungswahn und das Problem der Kausalität. *Zeitschrift für Psychopathologie* **3**, 86–127.

Hoche, A. (1934) In *Handbuch der gerichtlichen Psychiatrie*, 3rd edn. Berlin: Springer.

Homburger, A. (1926) *Vorlesungen über Psychopathologie der Kindesalters*. Berlin: Springer.

Hoppe, A. (1919) Wahn und Glaube. *Zeitschrift für die gesamte Neurologie und Psychiatrie* **51**, 124–207.

Iwanow-Smolensky, A. G. (1926) Über die Biogenese der Paranoia vom Standpunkte der modernen Grosshirn-Physiologie. *Allgemeine Zeitschrift für Psychiatrie* **85**, 240–56.

Jahrreiss, W. (1928) Störungen des Denkens. In *Handbuch der Geisteskrankheiten*, 1st part, ed. O. Bumke, pp. 530–99. Berlin: Springer.

Jaspers, K. (1923) *Allgemeine Psychopathologie*, 3rd edn. Berlin: Springer.

Jossmann, P. (1921) Das Problem der Überwertigkeit. *Zeitschrift für die gesamte Neurologie und Psychiatrie* **64**, 1–82.

Kahn, E. (1929) Über Wahnbildung. *Archiv für Psychiatrie und Nervenkrankheiten* **88**, 435–54.

Kant, O. (1927) Beiträge zur Paranoiaforschung. 1. Die objektive Realitätsbedeutung des Wahns. *Zeitschrift für die gesamte Neurologie und Psychiatrie* **108**, 625–44.

Kehrer, F. (1922) Der Fall Arnold. Studie zur neueren Paranoialehre. *Zeitschrift für die gesamte Neurologie und Psychiatrie* **74**, 155–217.

Knigge, F. (1935) Ein Beitrag zur Frage des primitiven Beziehungswahn. *Zeitschrift für die gesamte Neurologie und Psychiatrie* **153**, 622–8.

Kolle, K. (1931) Paraphrenia und Paranoia. *Fortschritte der Neurologie und Psychiatrie* **3**, 319–34.

Kraepelin, E. (1915) *Psychiatrie*, 8th edn. Leipzig: J. A. Barth.

Kraepelin, E. & Lange, J. (1927) *Psychiatrie*, 9th edn. Leipzig: J. A. Barth.

Kretschmer, E. (1918) *Der sensitive Beziehungswahn*, 2nd edn. Berlin: Springer.

Kronfeld, A. (1930) *Perspektiven der Seelenheilkunde*. Leipzig: G. Thieme.

Kunz, H. (1931) Die Grenze der psychopathologischen Wahninterpretationen. *Zeitschrift für die gesamte Neurologie und Psychiatrie* **35**, 671–715.

Lange, J. (1927) – see Kraepelin & Lange.

Langelüddeke, A. (1926) Zur Frage des sensitiven Beziehungswahnes. *Allegemeine Zeitschrift für Psychiatrie* **84**, 304–15.

Mayer-Gross, W. (1932) Paranoide und paraphrene Bilder. In *Handbuch der Geisteskrankheiten*, Spez. Teil 5, ed. O. Bumke. Berlin: Springer.

Mosbacher, F. W. (1931) Paraphrene Krankheitsbilder des Um- und Rückbildungsalters. *Archiv für Psychiatrie und Nervenkrankheiten* **93**, 46–83.

Neustadt, R. (1928) *Die Psychosen der Schwachsinnigen*. Berlin: Karger.

Reiss, E. (1921) Archaisch Denken der Schizophrenen. *Zentralblatt für die gesamte Neurologie und Psychiatrie* **35**, 432–67.

Scheid, W. (1937) Über Personenverkennung. *Zeitschrift für die gesamte Neurologie und Psychiatrie* **157**, 1–16.

Schilder, P. (1918) *Wahn und Erkenntnis*. Berlin: Springer.

Schneider, C. (1930) *Die Psychologie der Schizophrenen*. Leipzig: G. Thieme.

Schneider, K. (1931) *Psychopathologie im Grundriss*. Leipzig: G. Thieme.

Schulte, H. (1924) Versuch einer Theorie der paranoischen Eigenbeziehung und Wahnbildung. *Psychologische Forschung* **5**, 1–23.

Stoecker, W. (1919) Über Genese der Wahnideen, deren sekundäre Beeinflussung durch anderweitige psychische Faktoren. *Zeitschrift für die gesamte Neurologie und Psychiatrie* **49**, 94–158.

Storch, A. (1922) *Das archaisch-primitive Erleben und Denken der Schizophrenen*. Berlin: Springer.

Von Baeyer, W. (1932) Über konformen Wahn. *Zeitschrift für die gesamte Neurologie und Psychiatrie* **140**, 398–438.

Von Domarus, E. (1929) *Das Denken und seine Krankhaften Störungen*. Leipzig: Thieme.

Westerterp, M. (1924) Prozess und Entwicklung bei verschiedenen Paranoiatypen. *Zeitschrift für die gesamte Neurologie und Psychiatrie* **91**, 259–380.

Wetzel, A. (1922) Das Weltuntergangserlebnis in der Schizophrenie. *Zeitschrift für die gesamte Neurologie und Psychiatrie* **78i**, 403–28.

Wyrsch, J. (1935) Über Wahnbildung bei Alkoholdeliranten. *Allgemeine Zeitschrift für Psychiatrie* **103**, 67–75.

Zucker, K. (1939) Funktionsanalyse in der Schizophrenie. *Archiv für Psychiatrie und Nervenkrankheiten* **110**, 465–569.

Zutt, J. (1929) Die innere Haltung: eine psychologische Untersuchung und ihre Bedeutung für die Psychopathologie insbessondere im Bereich schizophrener Erkrankungen. *Monatsschrift für Psychiatrie und Neurologie* **73**, 330–83.

Werner Janzarik (1920–)

Werner Janzarik was born in Southern Germany and studied medicine in Würzburg. His psychiatric training was under Kurt Schneider in Heidelberg and after a period in Mainz he returned to Heidelberg in 1973 as professor of psychiatry and director of the psychiatric clinic. He is the editor of Nervenarzt, probably the most influential psychiatric journal in Germany and has written widely on the endogenous psychoses, including schizophrenia.

The present article differs from others in this volume, because it does not deal directly with a particular aspect of schizophrenia, but rather with the whole raison-d'être of descriptive psychopathology. It is based on a lecture delivered at a time when the anti-psychiatry movement was at its height in Germany and can be seen both as an apology and as a concise review of the trends in psychopathology during this century.

The crisis in psychopathology

W. Janzarik (1976)
(Die Krise der Psychopathologie. *Nervenarzt* **47**, 73–80)

This paper traces the development of psychopathological studies in German-speaking countries from the turn of this century to the present day. The crisis in which psychopathology finds itself is not a crisis of development, as Buehler considered was overtaking psychology in his day half a century ago, but rather a crisis of disinterest and insecurity in tune with the spirit of modern times. The purpose of this paper is to point out that the study of psychopathology is still as relevant as ever, in a field where all the major conditions are not scientifically defined disease entities, but exclusively psychopathologically defined syndromes. Furthermore, truly effective psychiatric treatment can never be developed until definitive psychopathological entities are established.

Fifty years ago Karl Buehler, a psychologist of some renown in the first half of the century, who taught in Vienna until his emigration, was asked to contribute an article on the state of psychology as part of a series called 'Studies on Kant'. As a point of departure Buehler began with the state of his discipline in the year 1890, when it was dominated by associationism, and then described the rapid development of a variety of different psychological schools of thought and their interactions at the beginning of this century. His book *The Crisis in Psychology*, based on this article, became a classic.

A report on the present state of psychopathology in German-speaking countries will likewise seem to describe a crisis. Here, too, the presentation of the contemporary state can take its point of departure from the revolution in the study of human sciences which took place at the turn of the century, and which still affects psychiatric thinking at the present time. We can then trace the various pathways and different directions by which psychopathology has arrived at its present state and consider how it finds itself in a crisis.

German psychopathology is orientated toward abnormal mental phenomena and is thus fundamental to clinical psychiatry. It has its origin in Karl Jaspers' book *General Psychopathology*, the first edition of which appeared in 1913. Jaspers was influenced by the revolution in psychology, the hermeneutical-understanding philosophy of Dilthey and Husserl's phenomenology. By careful attention to method, Jaspers succeeded in classifying psychopathological findings which had previously only existed in descriptive form. In so doing he formulated clear concepts and suggested appropriate topics for psychiatric research. Jaspers made use of Dilthey's twin concepts of 'understanding' and 'explaining'. He distinguished the concepts of 'process' and 'development' in psychiatric disorders, and had a profound influence on biological as well as psychopathological aspects of psychiatry. It was only with Jaspers that psychiatry achieved an awareness of method.

The science of descriptive psychopathology which he founded, which was then carried on by his pupils in the Heidelberg school, dominated psychiatric thinking in Germany for the next four decades. Jaspers himself left clinical psychiatry and devoted himself to philosophy, leaving his disciples, particularly Kurt Schneider, to apply his ideas to endogenous psychoses. Although Kurt Schneider remained unconvinced that manic-depressive psychosis and dementia praecox were 'diseases' rather than mere psychopathological entities, other members of the Heidelberg School – particularly Gruhle, Mayer-Gross and Wetzel – were more committed to an organic and a disease-orientated approach, following Kraepelin. At present, the continued influence of Jaspers' descriptive psychopathology can be seen in the work of Weitbrecht, Glatzel of Bonn and the Heidelberg paediatrician

Eggers. Kranz, Pauleikoff and Huber are others who developed some of his concepts under the direction of Kurt Schneider.

The next trend in psychopathology which we must consider is that developed by Kretschmer, best illustrated by his study of paranoid delusional formation in asthenic, irritable and sensitive personalities. He called such delusional states 'sensitive delusions of reference' (*Sensitiver Beziehungswahn*) and, following the teachings of Gaupp, tried to render understandable how such delusional states could develop independently of a schizophrenic process, through a combination of personality, environment and certain key experiences. Jaspers himself had been an examiner of Kretschmer's doctoral thesis and, although acknowledging its excellence, criticised him for ignoring the fundamental difference between understandable development and process in a psychosis. Ironically, it was this very aspect of the work which appealed to later psychiatrists. The Kraepelinian approach, emphasising the endogenous nature of psychosis, prevailed until the 1950s in German psychiatry and Kretschmer achieved his international reputation through his work on constitutional types and not through his psychopathological ideas. Since the Second World War, however, the ideas embodied in his notion of a *Sensitiver Beziehungswahn* have found wider application in German psychiatric writings. Even conservative psychiatrists are now prepared to consider the possibility of an environmental component in causing and not just precipitating a functional psychosis.

A third trend which we should acknowledge is the belated incorporation of the psychoanalytical teachings of Freud into the understanding of the psychoses. The older Heidelberg School of psychopathology had successfully employed its discipline of thinking and conceptual clarity to keep psychoanalysis out of German psychiatry. In Switzerland, through Eugen Bleuler, and in North America, through contributions from German-speaking emigrants from the Viennese circle and the Berlin Institute of Psychoanalysis, a synthesis between clinical psychiatry and psychoanalysis was attempted. Since the Second World War these ideas have been re-imported and can be found in the work of a number of German psychiatrists. This has resulted in a relaxation of the traditional German emphasis on genetics and endogenicity in psychotic development, and an appreciation of the role of family dynamics.

A fourth trend in psychopathology has been the influence of the science of anthropology. The two psychiatrists most committed to this approach were Straus and von Gebsattel. They wrote on the psychopathology of depression, compulsive phenomena and sexual perversion, taking as their standpoint the philosophical notions of Scheler on how an individual experiences life as a whole. More recently, Zutt has promoted the idea of an 'anthropological analysis' of psychiatric disorders.

The next trend to mention is the influence of existentialism, particularly the ideas of Heidegger, set out in his book *Being and Time* (*Sein und Zeit*). Ludwig Binswanger was the leading exponent of what was called 'existential analysis'. The object of this analysis was to gain new access to the world of a patient, who would then no longer be seen as subjectively isolated but as partaking of a certain existence, comprehensible in terms of his personal history and interpersonal relationships. Such ideas were at their zenith in Germany in the 1950s and 1960s. Zutt and Kulenkampf in Frankfurt, and von Baeyer, Kurt Schneider's successor in Heidelberg, promoted them avidly. They regarded a schizophrenic psychosis as an 'abnormal crisis' in a subject's life.

In the early 1960s in Frankfurt and Heidelberg there was yet another trend, a determined attempt to incorporate what was known about the social origins of psychosis into the framework of psychopathology. The roots of this trend were already present in Germany psychiatry, in the ideas of Kretschmer, but they were somewhat alien to tradition, and the new approach borrowed freely from British ideas. In my view, the development of a social psychiatric theory which would explain the concept of psychosis and its historical evolution is one of the most pressing tasks of present-day psychopathology.

From within psychology itself the most powerful influence on psychopathology has been *Gestalt* psychology, with the central concept that the sum of the component parts of perceptual experience is always less than the whole, the *Gestalt*. Although this psychological school was well developed between the two World Wars, by Wertheimer, Koehler and Koffka, the application of the ideas to abnormal phenomena only occurred after the Second World War. One application, to the study of personality and emotional disorder, was promoted in Germany by Welleck; another, on the consequences of brain damage and into the nature of schizophrenia, was pursued by Conrad. The essence of this approach is that, according to Conrad, aphasia and schizophrenia are both caused by a disintegration of a *Gestalt*; in the former condition it is language which suffers, in the latter it is perceptual unity. Matussek has, in recent years, extended Conrad's *Gestalt* analysis to explain how certain schizophrenic phenomena, hitherto regarded as abnormal beliefs, are in effect perceptual abnormalities.

At the present juncture in the history of our subject it is difficult to predict which contemporary intellectual trends are likely to exert an influence on psychopathological research in the future, bearing in mind the time it takes for new ideas to become manifest in the formulation of psychiatric theories. Current psychiatric practice presents a combination of pharmacotherapy and psychoanalytically supplemented social psychology. The occasional application of sociological role theory in problems encountered in psychopathology, as for instance in the analysis of the family background of schizophrenics, does not constitute a psychopathology based on sociology or social psychology. Similarly, structuralism as applied to linguistics and ethnology, although employed by Peters in the treatment of certain psychopathological disorders, has not produced anything that could be called a structuralistic psychopathology.

The renaissance of Marxism as a scientific method can be regarded as providing a critique of conventional psychiatric practice, but not of psychopathology itself. Until recently it was only the ritual incantations of Pavlov's first and second signalling systems that might be regarded as characteristic of a Marxist psychiatry. Notwithstanding the social psychiatric care of the population in well appointed out-patient clinics, the official psychiatry of the Socialist States bears, in its theoretical approach, such a conservative, Kraepelinian stamp that progressive young psychiatrists in the West would have to dismiss it as 'reactionary', 'capitalistic' and 'repressive'. There is, as yet, no Marxist psychopathology, perhaps because a method that is tailored to specific economic conditions cannot do justice to the subject.

The current crisis has been fuelled by the so-called anti-psychiatry movement, represented by the ideas of Basaglia, Cooper, Laing, Szasz and Foudraine. In its practical implications it owes much to the therapeutic community movement initiated by Maxwell Jones in Britain. Its theoretical origins can be traced in North American family research into schizophrenia. Szasz branded the concept of mental illness a 'myth', which served the purpose of excluding subjects who could not adapt to the questionable norms of an alienated society. In France, Britain and North America, these ideas are on the wane. Indeed, in France there is an anti-anti-psychiatry movement. In Germany, however, such ideas are still current. Take, for example, a comment made on the recent appointment to the vacant Chair of Psychiatry at Heidelberg:

> Heidelberg Psychiatry badly needed to take the opportunity of freeing itself at last from its inglorious past as the breeding ground of Psychopathology.

In spite of all the irritation caused by many an anti-psychiatrist in his naive arrogance, the psychopathologist is not without some sympathy as he notes the determination with which the nineteenth century biological disease concept in the case of the endogenous psychoses is called into question.

Alongside such philosophical, psychological and sociological influences, we must also consider the relationship between psychopathology and the biological sciences. It was the advent of effective biological treatments that forced psychiatrists to evaluate and measure various aspects of their clinical practice. This affected the field of psychopathology in two ways. Some psychiatrists, notably Heimann in Tübingen and Wieck in Erlangen, have tried to correlate traditional psychopathological findings with biological markers, what Wieck calls 'psychopathometry'. Others, notably Helmchen and Hippius, have tested empirical psychopathological groupings against the criteria of clinical relevance or the effectiveness of a particular therapeutic agent. It might appear from this that psychopathology is being increasingly subordinated to the biological approach, and that there is a danger that present-day psychology will be dominated, as in the late nineteenth century, by a neurophysiological version of associationism. In my view, this is not likely to happen, because of the very nature of the subject. One must recognise the existential and social dimensions of existence, and appreciate that psychotic experience cannot be reliably quantified.

A final influence, from amongst the biological sciences, is comparative behaviour research. Bilz pointed out the relevance of such findings for psychopathology, and Ploog has tried to confirm experimentally ideas such as that abnormal affective states, psychoses and degenerative conditions release inborn forms of behaviour. Such notions are reminiscent of Hughlings Jackson's levels of dissolution, which have periodically influenced the work of leading German psychiatrists, including Kraepelin.

These then are the major pathways which German psychopathology has taken. There is probably a personal bias in my selection, and each is presented rather briefly. What then is the current state of the discipline and what is the nature of its crisis? When Buehler spoke in 1926 of a crisis in psychology it was not, according to him, a crisis of decay and decline, but rather one of growth caused by a plethora and confusion of new ideas and methods. A review of all the modern trends in psychiatric research and practice could well arrive at the same conclusion. We are not concerned here with psychiatry as such, but with the difficulties of a specialised yet centrally orientated discipline which is developing its own methodology. The crisis of psychopathology thus defined is, at least at first sight, of depressing banality. It is the crisis of indifference, of resignation and of uncertainty, in an area of research that is in danger of slipping into a scientific no-man's-land because its major findings cannot be expressed in tables or in computer language.

There have been critical situations before. Around the year 1933 political ideology and violence erupted into the universities and paralysed academic life. About the same time there was a dawning in psychiatry of effective somatic therapies, obscure as they may have been in their mode of action. Scientific activity therefore withdrew into the therapeutic sector, it was impossible to justify the existence of a discipline which was regarded as useless by the anti-human spirit of the time. Psychotherapeutic research was paralysed. The blossoming of German psychopathology after the Second World War may be understood as a reaction to the decline brought about by political indoctrination and a pragmatism that was orientated towards therapy. It should, of course, not be overlooked that ever since the birth of clinical psychiatry at the beginning of the nineteenth century the major innovations have derived their incentive from therapeutic practice and fundamental changes in the management of psychiatric patients. When the empirical results of the newly introduced range of pharmacological treatments had been exhaustively discussed one might have expected a revival of interest in psychopathology, which in the meantime had again been relegated to the periphery. It never happened, and the lack of interest has, if anything, been accentuated. Psychopathology has become an idle pursuit without, to use a current phrase, 'social relevance'.

The cause of this decline is deeper than the simple triumph of therapeutic empiricism over theoretical examination and interpretation of the nature of psychiatric disorders. Present-day psychiatry finds itself at the mercy of forces created by the restructuring of an industrial society which has come to the limits of its demographic and technical expansion. Superficially, the crisis of psychopathology may appear unimportant. Beneath the surface, however, and in a way not seen in any other medical discipline, psychiatry is now failing to recognise its dependence on social change and the consequent need for a fundamental reorientation of its role and value. Kisker, for example, regards the problem faced by psychiatrists as a decision whether to resign oneself to the role of caretaker of institutionalised psychotics or to become a psychiatrist of society. He suggests that we should not play politics with psychiatry, but rather make politics work for our discipline.

If this prognosis is accurate then the psychiatrist will not be asked whether he likes his political role or not. He will have to accept it as a matter of fact. If he accepts it he will function as a social psychiatrist, exploiting those signs of the times which are favourable to his cause and engaging in politics on behalf of psychiatry. If he finds the political implications of social engineering unacceptable, then he will have to content himself with the limited role of clinical psychiatrist. Perhaps, in a 'universal psychiatry' of the future, he will even be surprised at what is expected of his old-fashioned private medical role, in spite of his preoccupation with group norms and in spite of the criminal values which will then be attached to certain individual deviations even in non-socialist countries. As psychopathologist he will have to have the courage to be a spoilsport who refuses to accept the limitation of psychiatry to its therapeutic role. With respect to psychiatry as a whole he will have to be a pluralist if he does not wish to narrow the range of his research and interests. His own personal interest in the phenomena of illness and experience will be too impractical and socially irrelevant, and he will find himself in opposition to the spirit of the times, attract hostility and find himself tempted to resign or escape into a more 'useful' or at least more socially acceptable activity.

Since psychology and sociology have become too dry and brittle as a result of their enslavement to statistical mathematics, the young are turning to the therapeutic medium of social psychiatric action. This is a new generation to whom pluralism even in science is meaningless, as it has not experienced the monotony of dictated thinking under the group terror of the National Socialist Peoples Community, nor the liberation therefrom. It is a generation which in the last analysis cannot be denied the right to despise feeble contemplation of its own activities and their consequences and which has not yet appreciated the meaning of historical enquiry. It is just to such a generation that psychopathological strivings seem hopelessly antiquated. Anyone who is afraid to be out of sympathy with the new generation and to fall behind as an old-fashioned outsider should not concern himself with psychopathological research.

It might seem an idle exercise to search for a way of resolving this crisis of psychopathology. It is not possible to halt the waves which mark the history of a science. One can only watch, and with a little experience attempt to predict the fluctuations and avoid being carried away. A science must be free to form hypotheses, to prove and disprove them, and to take into account its historical roots. For all the futuristic visions of psychiatry as a socio-psychological science of engineering and of the 'sociatrist' who runs it, the endogenous psychoses will continue to remain their central theoretical problem. It is no coincidence that present day paperback and popular psychiatry concerns itself nearly exclusively with schizophrenia, which after all makes up only a part of the endogenous psychoses and certainly only a fraction of the clinical material of psychiatry. And yet the purveyors of this kind of psychiatry think that they are embracing the whole of the subject in their critical polemics. Ironically, they are forgetting that schizophrenia and other endogenous psychoses are only psychopathological conventions. They may even be successful in their therapeutic endeavours within this framework, but they cannot maintain that they have the status of a scientist without knowing anything of the origins and methods of psychopathology.

The psychiatrist should not be restricted to the role apportioned to him by the social trends of the day, nor to some fashionable aspect of his subject, but he should be allowed to exercise the pluralism of his science. He should be given opportunities for therapeutic activity, and be forgiven when his work is uncritically accorded popular acclaim. But he should also be granted the freedom as psychopathologist to reflect on his activities and on the subject matter of his activities, and to strive for understanding in the obscurity of psychiatric experience.

II

French-language contributions

Philippe Chaslin (1857–1923)

Philippe Chaslin was born in Paris. His first love was mathematics and he was only persuaded to take up medicine by his grandfather who was a celebrated physician. He became senior psychiatrist at the Bicêtre Hospital in Paris and then at the Salpêtrière. A retiring bachelor, devoted to his mother and to his profession, he was an avid collector of books and knowledgeable about avant-garde poetry.

His psychiatric writings are marked by an aversion for conventional disease categories. He wrote about the influence of the dream in the content of delirious experience and about the role of primitive thinking in confusional states. His chief work, *Elements of Semiology and Clinical Mental Conditions* (1912), from which the present extract is taken, reflects his unconventional anti-organic stance. Nevertheless, his descriptions of *'Les folies discordantes'* is remarkably similar to that of Bleuler's schizophrenia published only a year before. The extract is chosen mainly to illustrate the remarkable convergence of European psychiatric ideas in the first decade of this century, despite the dissimilar backgrounds of the clinicians.

Discordant insanity

P. Chaslin (1912)

(Chapter 13, Groupe provisoire des folies discordantes, of *Eléments de Sémiologie et Clinique Mentales*. Asselin et Houzeau: Paris)

One can distinguish three principal types of discordant insanity in the early stages, although by the time dementia has supervened these distinctions become blurred. There is also a fourth type, which I call verbal insanity. The four types are: hebephrenia (which appears to be a mixed type); paranoid insanity (delusional insanity, previously called dementia paranoides); verbal insanity; and motor insanity or catatonia.

The word 'type' has the advantage that it has no precise nosological meaning. It is uncertain whether these types, although they have in common the general symptom of discordance, are several forms of the same disorder or constitute distinct conditions.

Hebephrenia

Attenuated form of hebephrenia. This is the most frequent form of hebephrenia, the one in which the attenuation of symptoms renders the diagnosis uncertain for long periods.

Case-history:
A boy of 14, with a family history of psychiatric disorder, became apathetic, lazy and inattentive. He was unable to continue his studies, and passed his days doing nothing other than playing with his sister's dolls. His intelligence and memory were unaffected, but he showed no interest in anything except childish games. He showed one of the most characteristic features of discordant insanity: non-coherence or discordance between different mental functions. While the boy was still capable of intellectual activity, he had lost all desire, wish and initiative to achieve anything. He was like a steam-engine without power, as if it had run out of fuel. The strange fashion in which he played with the dolls can be regarded as a form of eccentricity with regression. Despite the poor prognostic signs his condition remitted and he managed to pass one of his examinations, but his subsequent fate is unknown.

Hebephrenia. The following case illustrates many of the features of this type.

Case-history:
The patient was a milliner aged 20 who was brought to the Salpêtrière by her mother. The latter reported: 'My daughter has changed a lot over the past two years. She used to be a skilled milliner, but now she does nothing. Two years ago she was sent to a new workshop and from that time she suddenly changed. No one else in our family has had anything like this. She didn't have any fits as a baby but was always very nervous; she would cry at the smallest thing, was always a little aggressive but could be kind too, and was jealous of her brother and sister. Then she became so fearful that she had to sleep with me. The first real sign of anything seriously wrong was one evening when she said: "Come and feel my stomach. It's not moving. I'm going to die. Come here, mummy and daddy. Let me kiss you." Since then, the fear of dying hasn't left her. Now, all she does all day long is fiddle about with cards, papers or ribbons, or else she just sits doing nothing . . . Every evening she pretends that she has been working all day and earning three francs a day. This is completely untrue. She even says that she is supporting *us* and calls us lazy. She detests my husband and me, says that we are making a martyr of her and treats me cruelly. She won't talk to us, thinks we're inferior to her, and if we touch her she says that we are making her dirty. In fact, she is letting herself go, neglecting herself and has terrible table manners. She throws her shoes and skirts in the fire. Despite all this she knows what is going on and there is nothing wrong with her memory. She feels she is going mad, or so she says. At one time she wanted to kill herself, to jump in the Seine, but never did anything, and after six months the

idea passed off. This was about a year ago. She seems fed up with everything, to the point that she can't even be bothered to sleep. I don't know if she sleeps or not. I've heard her talking to herself at night. Her willpower and good spirits have completely left her. Sometimes she says that her hands won't work any more, or that her feet have ceased functioning . . .'

In summary, the patient was a young woman with an abnormal childhood whose condition began suddenly with hypochondriacal ideas, paranoid ideas and non-systematised grandiose ideas. There were bizarre sensations, disorganised behaviour, fugues, suicidal tendencies, indifference alternating with hostility, fear of dying, bouts of anxiety, lying, a mocking smile and a partial awareness of her situation. The illness had been present for about two years. She had, in effect, a veritable 'salad' of symptoms which justifies the term discordant insanity. On direct mental state examination, however, there was remarkably little to find . . .

Paranoid insanity (dementia paranoides of Kraepelin)

This type of illness is not as common as hebephrenia. The following case illustrates the typical features of paranoid insanity.

Case-history:
The patient was a woman who presented with an incoherent set of delusions to which she was singularly indifferent. They were full of incredible contradictions and absurdities, and were accompanied by outbursts of excitement, laughter and gestures which bore no relationship to and often contradicted the ideas which she was expressing. The excitement was more marked at the onset of her condition and tended to occur in the presence of people whom she believed were harming her. At such times she could become violent. Some of the extravagant statements included the following:
'I am pregnant with Jesus Christ in my mind, my heart and my womb. I am the mistress of thirty Kings as well as Napoleon. My divorce was passed by all the churches. I went to the High Court and was told that I wasn't mad. I died of chickenpox and one of the Bourbon family came and got me out of the cemetery. I wanted to eat asparagus but they made me eat filth. Every night I'm buried alive; I'm cut up into pieces and Kings come and sleep with me while I'm hypnotised . . .'

In this case, the prominence of the delusions places it alongside other systematised paranoid insanity (the 'paranoia' of other authors). However, it differs from these other delusional states in that the delusions are not only polymorphous but also incoherent and absurd, and this incoherence is not merely a function of excitement but persists even when the patient is in a cold unemotional frame of mind. Except at the onset of her illness the patient has been emotionally indifferent the whole time and all her natural feelings, such as maternal love, have disappeared. It is only her persecutory ideas which now raise any emotion. The main features of her condition are the rapid dissociation between ideas and emotion, secondary stereotypies, discordance, the preservation of memory even after five years, and an absurd, polymorphous, extravagant and incoherent set of delusions. This is characteristic of paranoid insanity, exhibited in pure form by this case, which merits the label 'schizophrenia' which certain authors have given it. Dementia paranoides, another term sometimes used, takes account of the content of the delusions but fails to convey the fact that intelligence is partially preserved . . .

Discordant verbal insanity

In addition to discordant delusional or paranoid insanity, discussed above, there is a separate type characterised by an extraordinary verbal incoherence without any true delusions. It is not entirely clear whether the paranoid and verbal types should be separated, because one could argue that the former is not really a disorder of belief but of verbal expression. Be that as it may, the following is a case of discordant verbal insanity whose features are so characteristic as to justify its separation from the other types.

> *Case-history:*
> The patient was a man aged 42 when he was admitted to the Bicêtre hospital. He had been regarded as very intelligent up to the age of 16, when he visited England to learn the language and study business methods. On his return to France he began to work as an employee in a commercial firm. He then began to stay away from work without explanation and to mislay letters which he had been asked to post. He had outbursts of excitement when he would throw things through the window. He would hit his mother without apparently recognising her. In addition, there were periods of mutism during which he would remain for hours in front of the fire, his head in his hands. His first admission to hospital had been at this period when he lost consciousness while visiting Beauvais cathedral. He was said to have been unconscious for 15 hours. He then did his military service, but spent most of it in and out of hospital with nervous complaints. After

his discharge he was admitted to a psychiatric hospital and from then on he has been completely incoherent in his speech. Whenever his mother visits him he talks fairly normally at first, asks sensible questions about his relatives, but after a few minutes he begins to ramble again.

On examination he always presents the same picture. Grey-haired, small, active and perpetually moving about, he is generally to be seen talking to himself, even at night, and does not appear demented. He has an intelligent-looking face and always addresses an interlocutor politely. He looks after himself and is well adjusted to asylum life. He keeps himself clean, exhibits good table manners, but rarely talks to his neighbours. As for his relationship with the nurses, they have to put up with his constant demands for tobacco. He is indifferent to visits from outsiders, although he always receives his mother kindly. He has nothing to occupy his time; he plays no games and does not join in with the other patients, spending the whole day walking about.

At interview, he is usually co-operative and gives the impression of being interested in the exchange. His eyes light up, he smiles and makes gestures underlining some of the strange phrases which he emits. Here is a sample of conversation:

Patient:	*Psychiatrist:*
'Hallo, how are you?	How are you?
Have you come to fetch me?	I just want to talk for a while
He won't give me any tobacco	Who won't?
The Government	What's your complaint?
Every month, a packet worth six sous arrives. It's not enough, so I wonder if you could give me some	What do you smoke?
Cigarettes. I keep them in my pocket. Why don't you give me some?	I haven't got any. How long have you been here?
For centuries. How long is it?	I'm asking you
I don't know how many years. They pass so quickly	Do you know today's date?
I don't bother with dates. We must be in the year 1908 or 1909	1908. What month?
I don't know, I live like a mole	I understand you speak English well?
Yes, but English, I can't say a word. It is as if you changed climate. Someone's changing	

me. *Boalabese*, it is a lake of
azene. I see myself in the sea, it
is the sea, it is made of cotton
and wool.   Are we talking of your travels!
It's the sea in any case   Have you been to South
                                               America?
No   In Alaska then?
Yes. We will see that later. I'm
going to get a job as a veteran
"aide de camp"   What is that?
It's your business. It's the sea in
simée looking at itself in a sea,
if I bother about your affairs.
Aide de camp, it is the sea
simée; the azene, you send it for
a walk, always running, even
it lives somewhere, if you
make clay run it will live in the
azene'

Discordant motor insanity, catatonia

Motor phenomena can so dominate the clinical picture in some patients
that a particular form of insanity is thereby established. Borrowing
Kahlbaum's term I shall designate this type as catatonia. The following
patient illustrates the condition.

Case history:
The patient was a man of 32 when admitted to the Bicêtre. Father was
rheumatic and syphilitic and his mother intelligent and active, but the
victim of unfortunate circumstances. The patient completed his secondary education but left school without passing examinations and
followed no career. He was a bank employee for a few months and
married at the age of 29. He was subject to frequent falls and after
reading books about hypnosis began to believe, at the age of 31, that
his uncle was making him fall by the power of suggestion. At the same
time he developed ideas of grandeur, believing that his wife was of
noble birth . . . From his admission in 1903 until the end of 1906 the
only data recorded were brief comments on his mental state and a
weight chart. One of these comments stated that the patient 'is
affected by manic excitement, disordered ideas and behaviour, rambl-
ing speech; ideas of persecution, of poisoning, of grandeur and of
mysticism; a feeling that he must redeem the sins of mankind; and a

tendency to sing, shouting, whistling, violent outbursts, insomnia, and refusal of food . . .'.

In February 1907 he was adopting cataleptic attitudes. He would maintain his arms for a long time in any position that they were placed. He would stay for an entire half-day with his arms outstretched, the palm of his hand turned upwards and his head and eyes facing the wall . . .

In September 1908 he would recite litanies in a singsong and declamatory fashion: 'Monsieur Vincent – five years; *embaude* – five years; enfer (Hell) – ten years; *emmarmet* – ten years; *emmar* – ten years; *emcatholique* – ten years . . .'.

In summary, his childhood and adolescence were abnormal and marked by extreme laziness. The onset of his condition was heralded by neurasthenic symptoms, followed by delusions of persecution and grandeur. There was intermittent agitation and, in the early period of his admission, he seemed to have preserved his intelligence. Later he engaged in declamatory litanies, showed catatonic stupor and developed secondary disabilities from his abnormal postures. At this stage, too, he had become indifferent to his surroundings, and he would alternate between negativism and suggestibility; stereotypies and neologisms became more frequent.

Discussion

Discordance and discordant insanity. Is each of the types described under the general title of discordant insanity a separate form of insanity or only a particular form of the same illness? Is the link between these types – the discordance – sufficient to categorise them as one form of insanity? Clinical observations do not provide an answer at present and I do not intend to construct a nosological system. The term 'clinical type' is intended to be non-committal.

Whatever the situation may be, clinically there seems to be a link between the various types. It appears as if there are transitions between them, and that one can identify approximately three phases – the onset, the established state, and the terminal stage.

It was Kraepelin who joined together the hebephrenia of Hecker and Kahlbaum, the catatonia of Kahlbaum and dementia paranoides under the rubric of 'dementia praecox'. There is also the question of systematised hallucinatory insanity, which I believe is distinct from these and which I shall keep separate.

Dementia in discordant insanity. The term 'dementia praecox' chosen by Kraepelin is unfortunate because, as we have seen, dementia only supervenes after many years. Bleuler used the word 'schizophrenia' to characterise this type of insanity whereas I prefer the term 'discordant insanity', which reflects the intrapsychic ataxia noted by Stransky and the intrapsychic dysharmony observed by Urstein. Dementia, even if it occurs, does not appear to be very pronounced; it is more like the end stage of the systematised insanities where, more often than not, it does not occur at all or is very mild. Patients suffering from 'dementia praecox' are always less demented than they appear. If the term 'dementia praecox' is taken to mean an early onset to the condition, this is also inappropriate because many patients develop their illness in later life, in middle age or even old age, and one finds such paradoxical terms as 'late onset dementia praecox' or 'late onset catatonia' in the literature . . .

Conclusions

Discordant insanity has as its main characteristic a discordance or dysharmony between symptoms, which therefore appear as if they had no connection with one another. Klippel found organic changes in the nervous system in some of these cases. If this is true of all cases of all types then we will be able to regard discordant insanity as having a known cause. At the present time, however, this is not certain.

Generally, there is a family history of psychiatric disorder and, often, the patient demonstrated abnormal features in childhood.

There are four principal types of discordant insanity: hebephrenia and attenuated hebephrenia; paranoid insanity; verbal insanity; and catatonia. Epileptic fits can occur in any of these types. The development of the condition may be intermittent particularly in hebephrenia and catatonia. The outcome is grave, as it is doubtful whether full remission ever occurs, although there may be some improvement.

There is no effective treatment.

Hebephrenia. The *onset* is between 8 and 25 years of age, or at the very latest 30; some authors place the upper limit as even later. The disorder can commence slowly, quickly or insidiously.

The *first symptoms* are laziness, indifference, slowness at work, conflicts with others, outbursts of anger and periods of sadness; in short, there is a change in personality. Sometimes there are periods of unexplained excitement, fugues, tics, outbursts of laughter, grimacing, bizarre attitudes, infantile behaviour, vague delusional ideas and inexplicable nocturnal or day-time fears. Excessive masturbation may occur. Complaints about the state of health are common. Hysterical seizures, migraine, neuralgia, anorexia, constipation, insomnia and nightmares may be prominent at this time. It is usually the school teacher who is the first to pick up a change in attitude, work performance or general appearance. These are first attributed to laziness and disobedience on the part of the pupil, whereas they are the first signs of the developing illness.

In the *established phase* there is an accentuation of all these phenomena, with each case presenting a slightly different pattern. In some patients depression and sadness may be prominent: there may be delusional ideas with a vague persecutory content, suicidal tendencies, anxiety, impotence, or difficulties in movement, thinking or acting. Excitement and pressure of speech may stand out along with agitation, pseudomania, anger, motiveless outbursts of laughter, infantile behaviour, silly jokes, tics, stereotyped and extravagant movements, disorganised and bizarre writing, idiosyncratic use of language, fugues and anti-social incidents. Other patients may show mainly persecutory ideas, with or without hallucinations. Others may have grandiose ideas. All these phenomena usually have a strange and disorganised appearance. More remarkable is the fact that they are quite superficial in the position they hold in the patient's mind. Underneath there is usually a complete indifference or apathy which is only interrupted by occasional bouts of catatonia with excitement, stupor or negativism. At the same time intelligence, memory, judgement and sometimes attention are preserved to a surprising degree. In short, intelligence remains intact, at least for lengthy periods, but the patient no longer makes use of it, as he does not work and does virtually nothing other than engage in infantile or automatic acts. The patient's attitude sometimes makes one think that he is simulating insanity, making fun of the interviewer or acting a part. His strange movements, his often contradictory facial expression, his ironic smiles and laughter, his grimacing and his flights of fancy all contribute to this impression . . .

In the *demented phase* there is intellectual impairment of varying degrees. The symptoms of the earlier phases lose their distinctness and become stereotyped. The patient remains standing, lying or sprawled out in a corner, dirty and slovenly. Activity is restricted to gobbling up food. Life seems purely vegetative and automatic, although one is sometimes surprised to find sparks of intelligence beneath this envelope of dementia. Another curious feature of the condition is the preservation, in some cases, of an intelligent facial expression. At this stage the patient is fit only for simple tasks; only a few ever regain their former activity or return to society, and even these rare cases are not cured, only improved.

Attenuated hebephrenia resembles neurasthenia in some ways, but the extreme indifference and pathological laziness should make one suspect the former. Bizarre gestures, idiosyncratic and fleeting interest in things, tics, grimaces, outbursts of laughter and infantile preoccupations all occur, but in a more sketchy fashion than in fully developed hebephrenia.

The *differential diagnosis* includes neurasthenia (rare in childhood and often concealed); obsessional neurosis – which may precede hebephrenia, but there is no indifference, no personality change and no loss of insight; tics and chorea, distinguished by the characteristic movements; tuberculous meningitis, where there are signs of meningitis; epileptic dementia, predominantly a loss of intelligence with slowness and emotional outbursts; general paralysis of the insane and cerebral syphilis, identified by physical signs and lumbar puncture; epileptic confusional states, with a history of fits; and psychopathic states which may precede hebephrenia but without movement disorder or delusions. Other conditions which may be mistaken for hebephrenia include: acute organic psychosis, with transient disturbance of intellectual functions; epileptic psychosis, usually short-lived and with a history of fits; mania, where there is a more widespread involvement of mental functions and never as a cause of stereotypes or mannerisms; depression, rare in late childhood and distinguished by the genuine emotional pain that one witnesses; chronic systematised insanity [paranoia – Tr.], identified by the systematised delusions, the coherence of all the phenomena, suspiciousness and the lack of indifference – indeed one usually finds the opposite, an intense preoccupation with the symptoms; acute insanity, characterised by a polymorphous but incoherent pattern to the delusions; and hysteria, where there is marked suggestibility, convulsive attacks of a special type and altered consciousness.

Paranoid insanity. This usually begins in early adulthood rather than childhood, and sometimes begins in middle age.

Its *onset* is usually abrupt, with several different types of delusional ideas with or without hallucinations. The ideas may concern persecution, grandeur, hypochondria, nihilistic notions, bodily change or inventive topics. They may be accompanied by depression, anxiety, agitation or rapture. Intelligence appears intact at this stage.

In the *next phase* emotional reactions disappear and the delusions become extravagant, absurd, changeable, diffuse and contradictory. There is usually indifference or euphoria, an ironic facial expression, incoherent speech, preserved memory and intelligence, and catatonic signs . . .

Finally, dementia of varying severity supervenes after several months or years.

The differential diagnosis includes all those conditions which give rise to incoherent delusions: delirium tremens, infectious delirium, epileptic psychosis, general paralysis, hallucinatory delusional states (where the hallucinations dominate the picture), chronic systematised insanity, and acute insanity.

Discordant verbal insanity. This is rare. In pure forms, after an initial phase which is similar in all respects to the early stages of the other types, the clinical picture changes and becomes dominated by completely incoherent language. Neologisms are frequent and, although words are expressed with normal intonation and appropriate smiles or gestures, their meaning is completely incomprehensible. Patients indulge in dialogues and monologues, uttered with normal facial expression but accompanied by total indifference. It seems as if intelligence is less affected than language itself, and that the thought disorder may stem from this disorder of language.

The differential diagnosis lies between all these conditions which cause incoherent language. Most of them, however, are immediately eliminated because they do not produce such an abundance of neologisms. The main problem is to distinguish discordant verbal insanity from cases of chronic systematised insanity where there is a secret, symbolic language.

Catatonia. The onset may be similar to that of the other types or the final episode itself may be a catatonic attack . . . During a period of stupor the patient usually retains normal attention and memory, but appears unable to use them to engage in any intellectual task, because of indifference and apathy. Once he has started a task, however, there appears to be no difficulty, even in carrying out certain movements. The slowing down of ideas does not come about through inhibition. The slowness is apparent even before a response or action and stems from a mechanism which we can call 'association by contrast'. It was this mechanism which Kraepelin called *Sperrung* (blocking) as opposed to *Hemmung* (inhibition).

There are often physical signs to be seen: unequal pupils, dilated pupils, exaggerated reflexes, excessive salivation . . .

The condition may last a considerable time until dementia supervenes.

The differential diagnosis includes other conditions which produce catatonic features, although in these cases the catatonic signs are transient and incomplete: infectious delirium and dementia, traumatic and epileptic psychoses, general paralysis, cerebral tumour, idiocy, depression and hysteria.

Ernest Dupré (1862–1921)

Ernest Dupré was born in Marseilles but spent most of his life in Paris. His father became a teacher of rhetoric in a Parisian grammar school. After qualifying as a physician he studied general medicine for several years and then chose to specialise in psychiatry. He became the director of a hospital for the criminally insane and most of his publications reflect his interest in forensic psychiatry.

During the First World War he campaigned for more adequate psychiatric services for the French soldiers and described the frequent occurrence of a neurotic reaction among combatants, which one of his pupils termed 'Dupré's disease'. Dupré was a cultured man who tried, in his writings, to accommodate the 19th century views of Morel and Magnan on 'degenerates' with more enlightened and psychological notions of how disturbed imagination and emotional disorder could lead to antisocial behaviour.

Dupré is celebrated for inventing the term 'mythomania' – a tendency in some people to fabricate the events of their life. The article selected here, which he wrote with Logre, is an attempt to explain how this mythomanic tendency could lead to the development of a psychosis.

Jean Logre (1883–1963)

Jean Logre was born in Lisieux in Normandy. He studied medicine in Paris and then turned to psychiatry, first as a pupil and then as a collaborator with Dupré. He was appointed director of the hospital for the criminally insane in Paris on the death of de Clérambault.

Logre was a cultured man, an expert on Latin verse, who was respected by the French psychoanalytical school. He wrote a comprehensive textbook of psychiatry. The article translated here illustrates his interest in forensic and nosological issues.

Confabulatory delusional states
E. Dupré and J. Logre (1911)
(Les délires d'imagination, *Encéphale* **6a**, 209–32)

Introduction

In 1910 we introduced the term 'confabulatory delusional states' to designate those psychiatric conditions where there was a selective disorder of the faculty of creative imagination. They are the result of a heightened creative activity, leading to the spontaneous association of images and ideas into new combinations. These inventive constructions, which correspond to some extent with reality, represent the subjective and autogenic products of the mind. Their content expresses the personal inclinations of the subject, and their complexity is a function of the strength and mobility of a subject's psychological make-up. Although imagination has a role in the formation of all delusions, it is never so exclusively involved as in those states that we are considering here. In other cases the crucial element in the formation of a delusion is an error in the way a subject views the world, or a perceptual disorder, or a pathological way of reasoning.

A more detailed comparison of the probable origin of various delusional states will serve to highlight what we regard as the characteristic feature of these confabulatory states.

In hallucinatory delusional states, whether acute (toxic delirium, delirium tremens, bouffées délirantes) or chronic (the hallucinatory psychoses described by Séglas and Cotard, the hallucinoses of Dupré), the predominant disorder is one of perception. The subject regards as real perceptions what are in effect subjective products of his mind. At the same time the perceptual disorder determines the content of the delusion by presenting the material to be incorporated. In pure hallucinatory states a patient may embroider what he regards as a genuine event in the outside world, but such interpretations are natural and logical. The position is sometimes complicated by the fact that patients may have an associated confusional state, and their interpretations may appear pathological for this reason, but the primary origin of any delusion is the perceptual disorder, and it is not necessary to introduce a disorder of reasoning or imagination to explain its development. In classic hallucinatory delusional states one may find abundant and absurd interpretations which go beyond what should be natural interpretations of their hallucinations; nevertheless, even in these cases the hallucination always plays a major role.

In misinterpretative delusional states one assumes that the disorder arises at a more advanced stage along the chain of operations which run from simple perception to states of belief and certainty. The error made by someone with hallucinations is in the sphere of perception. The error of a misinterpretation is in the sphere of logic, as in this case perception is not affected. The problem is not one of registering information, but of appreciating it, recognising its links with other phenomena and establishing its relative importance and significance, in short, in its interpretation. The powers of argument, although not lacking in strength, are qualitatively affected. Subjects afflicted by this condition are worried by what they see, and have a continual need to fit it all together. They feel obliged to do this and, although they are remarkably skilled in arriving at subtle conclusions, these are in fact tendentious, specious and false. The plethora of arguments at their command hides, in reality, an impoverished logic. Their delusions reflect a dialectic distorted by a dominant emotion. Such patients proceed by induction and deduction; in short, by inference.

Those subjects affected by a confabulatory delusional state, on the other hand, are not at all worried by what they see in the outside world; nor do they feel an urge to embark on elaborate logical proofs of what is there. Instead they express ideas or recount stories without caring whether they conform with reality. Reality to them is their own association of ideas and subjective creations, which they invest with all the characteristics of objectivity. They proceed by intuition, auto-suggestion and invention. The point of departure for their mistaken view of the world is not an idea about some external event, exact or inexact, or a false way of reasoning, or a false perception, but a fiction of endogenous origin, a subjective creation. Misinterpretation is a cognitive process, confabulation a poetic process.

In confabulatory delusional states certain events and emotions may act as a trigger, but even here misinterpretation and invention can be distinguished. Confabulatory delusional states do not arise from a sense of necessity or an examination of the logical consequence of an event. Ideas are not linked by formal rules but are more like scenes in a story, outside the operations of discursive thought; they spring up spontaneously. Even if the patient draws attention to the source of his observation, he does it in an episodic and casual manner. Reality merely furnishes his mind with a theme on which his imagination can work at its leisure, to provide variations and improvisations. If he does argue, it is not through any spontaneous urge to do so, but merely to counter the objections of others . . .

In subjects with a misinterpretative delusional state, belief cannot grow without the help of perceptions and logical operations; in confabulatory delusional states the belief is already present by virtue of the immediate evidence. There is also a real temperamental difference between subjects who rely on reasoning, who are prone to misinterpretations, and those who rely on intuition, who are prone to confabulations.

These distinctions between hallucinatory, misinterpretative and confabulatory delusional states, it should be stressed, are schematic and largely artificial. All have elements in common, and mixed states may occur . . .

The further development of a delusional system is determined by the same factors which gave rise to it in the first place. Delusions based on misinterpretations grow because the subject continually consolidates the system by noting further incidents and making further inferences. Delusions based on imagination are enriched by further fictions and their most distinctive feature is the richness of the creative imagination, particularly the tendency to fabricate in an extempore manner.

The tendency to alter reality, to lie and to fabricate, which one of us previously referred to as 'mythomania', derives from a 'disequilibrium in the imaginative faculty', and provides the basis for this condition. All 'mythomanic subjects', including children and mentally deficient individuals who often lie deliberately, are credulous and may come to believe their own stories. In confabulatory delusional states, however, there is, in addition, the setting up of a collection of systematic and more or less permanent beliefs, and this passes beyond what can be considered normal.

The development of the condition, in brief, can be regarded as a morbid exaggeration of a constitutional tendency towards 'mythomania'. In its pure form, however, the condition is rare, certainly less common than the pure forms of hallucinatory and misinterpretative delusional states . . . In clinical practice one often meets examples of 'simple fabrication', where fictional events are accepted as genuine, and various transitional states between these instances of a simple fabrication and the rare systematised confabulatory delusional states.

Another reason for its apparent rarity is the tendency among doctors to interrogate patients rather than to let them express their thoughts freely . . . In consequence some patients with a confabulatory delusional state appear to be suffering from a misinterpretative delusional state because they are compelled to justify every idea. In this way, some misinterpretative delusional states may represent, like hysteria, a collaborative effort on the part of doctor and patient.

Confabulatory delusional states can occur as a relatively pure condition, as a particular kind of paranoid or grandiose syndrome, associated with some other condition, or as an episode in the course of a variety of psychiatric disorders.

The following case, in which confabulatory delusions were seen in relative isolation, illustrates the condition. There were no hallucinations and hardly any misinterpretative elements.

Case history:

On 24th May 1908 the police brought to hospital a woman who gave her name as X and was about 25 years of age. She claimed to be a painter and the divorced wife of Mr K. She was accompanied by two children who, she said, were the offspring of her ex-husband and her own sister. She announced that this sister had died that very day. She had been brought to hospital following complaints to the police that she had been behaving and talking in an extravagant fashion.

For some time she had been moving from hotel to hotel in Paris, staying no more than three days in each, and leaving without paying her bill. She had taken taxis without paying her fare, and had told the police that she was the victim of numerous thefts, swindles and confidence tricks, and that she was related to several European royal families. On enquiry, it transpired that she was actually homeless and penniless.

She was transferred from hospital to prison to stand trial on the charge of fraud. More details about her behaviour prior to her arrest then emerged. For example, between 9th and 12th May she had stayed at the Hotel Chateau de Madrid at Neuilly-sur-Seine, where she had run up a bill of 443 francs and made several telephone calls to the British, German and Spanish ambassadors.

Her own account of her life was as follows: 'I don't know where I was born. I don't know who my parents were nor what nationality I am. I was married about seven years ago in Saint-Germain to a man called Mr K. and have been divorced for four years. My husband was instructed by my solicitor, Mr B., to pay me an alimony of 38,000 francs, but I received none of this. This is why I have got into debt. The two children who are with me, Suzanne aged 11 and Edward aged 9, are the children of my husband and my sister, Rosine, now dead. I was given custody of them after my divorce. I cannot explain the complaint of the taxi-driver, as I instructed him to get his fare from my solicitor Mr F. at 26 Rue d'Alger'.

When again questioned about her identity, she replied: 'My mother was travelling when I was born. She took me all over the place, Valparaiso, Cyprus, and two other places which I don't remember. I have 11 names. I was sent to school at Montmorency and Princess Mathilde paid for my education. A few months ago the King of Spain, whose portrait I painted, made me a member of the Bourbon family, and so today I am related to the Spanish royal family . . .'.

Her real background was eventually uncovered. She had indeed been married and divorced and her alimony had never been paid, but the years she mentioned were incorrect and the sum only involved 200 francs a month. Her two children were really her own. She continued to fabricate during her stay in prison; her son was the heir to the King of England; she had vast sums of money in the bank; important people were trying to rob her of this money. None of this was true. She remained in prison for five years and was then sent to an asylum, her inventions still unchanged.

Discussion

Her delusional state was remarkably free of any psychopathological element outside the sphere of confabulation. There were no hallucinations and few misinterpretations. This latter fact needs to be carefully examined, as there are several ways in which her inventions might be taken for misinterpretations. For example, it might be that she was remembering an event which she had misinterpreted at the time; or that she had a correct memory for a real event, but was now misinterpreting it – a retrospective misinterpretation; or that the incident mentioned by the subject did not correspond to any real event at all. In our view, the patient's inventions cannot be accounted for in either of the first two ways. It is not a question of misinterpretation in her case, but of retrospective fabrication. This phenomenon is sometimes referred to as an hallucination of memory, but in effect the disorder has more to do with imagination than memory. Her creative imagination was presenting its fabrications in the guise of memory, and she then believed that she remembered something. Memory itself has nothing intrinsically to do with her inventions. She merely has the *illusion* of a memory.

Mrs X. asserted that her husband owed her a substantial alimony, but a tribunal had ordered him to pay a monthly figure of only 200 francs. This is an exaggeration and distortion of the facts, an invention and not an inference. As with her other fabrications, it was as if she were telling a tale, one incident following another, and one anecdote suggesting a new one. Even the documents which she claimed to have in her possession were inventions. There was no fact or event which we can say that she had misinterpreted. There was only a fabrication of material proof, the exact opposite of what happens in misinterpretative states.

In some cases external incidents are not invented but merely used to justify original fabrications. For instance, the patient showed us a scar on her face which she claimed was the result of an assassin's attack.

The scar was in fact there, but had nothing to do with any assault on her person . . .

The patient can justifiably be regarded as a 'constitutional mythomanic'. Her real mother, who was finally traced, told us that her daughter had always had a 'rich imagination' which led her into trouble. One of us had previously listed the varieties of mythomania as malign or perverse, defensive, and conceited or indulgent. Our patient illustrates all three. She had pretensions to be an artist of note; she invented to protect herself and to satisfy her erotic and acquisitive nature; and she fabricated in a boastful way to show herself in the most favourable light.

We are particularly struck by the method by which such patients develop and embroider their themes. It is usually done in an extempore way, off the cuff, so to speak, in response to questions by the doctor. Thus, as noted earlier, the doctor participates in the inventions. Suggestibility and 'passive fabrication' go together with spontaneous invention and 'active fabrication'.

As each invented idea is produced, it is then registered as if it were an incontrovertible fact, inscribed, as it were, on a 'mythomanic dossier'. After a while, secondary interpretations and the guiding influence of emotional preoccupations then consolidate a complex system which constitutes the more or less permanent phase of a confabulatory delusional state.

It is worth considering the theme of the delusions as well as their mode of development and the abundance of their content. The incidents referred to are always rare, singular and extraordinary. They remind one of the scenes from romantic fiction or adventure stories. They portray events which are impossible and extreme. Patients talk of immense wealth, of princes and of kings. A woman is not only the mistress of some powerful person, she is the mistress of all the kings of Europe, and of Asia as well. Not content with possessing millions, they distribute them to everyone. In some ways the condition resembles general paralysis but, unlike the latter, inventive delusional states contain a strong element of persecution and complaint. One is reminded of Renan's observation that 'imagination has more links with desire than with fear' . . .

In their general structure these delusional states are remarkably complex and polymorphous. They are made up of the juxtaposition of a large number of themes which have in common elements of grandeur and persecution and a flavouring of erotic and political preoccupations.

Sometimes the multiplicity and incompatibility of their beliefs make the patient appear incoherent, but usually the logic behind them can be identified.

A further characteristic of the fabrications of our patient was the paradoxical combination of both sincerity and simulation, of naivety and duplicity. Mrs X. was a liar, a deceitful rogue, a joker and a hoaxer. But she was also a victim of her own tales, gained little profit from them, and eventually suffered by them. This occurs in nearly all cases and can be regarded as a 'deficit in the sense of verification and a distortion of the notion of reality'. This childish naivety, lack of judgement and absence of a critical sense are also seen in mentally deficient individuals.

Finally, one should note that the behaviour of patients with this condition accords with their inventions. Although their conversation often resembles that of a liar, their behaviour is undoubtedly that of a deluded person. As Bain noted, action is the ultimate criterion of belief. Mrs X. rented expensive flats which she could not inhabit, ran up debts which would only lead to imprisonment, wrote letters to kings, and telephoned ambassadors. And when her extravagant behaviour led to complaints and legal repercussions, she responded indignantly, demanded redress and believed herself to be an innocent victim.

Medicolegal considerations

The medicolegal consequences of this condition are, to a certain extent, its hallmarks.

The behaviour which brings the patients into conflict with the law is as varied and exuberant as their delusions. Their police dossier is as voluminous as their clinical file. The patients have usually written to innumerable people, and telephoned all kinds of officials. Their behaviour in this respect amounts to a veritable 'graphorrhoea'. The most characteristic features are the habit of bearing false testimony, claiming descent from a royal or noble family, fraud and vagrancy.

Bearing false testimony takes the form of accusing supposed persecutors with having committed certain acts. Our patient claimed to have documented evidence on such matters. Sometimes patients mention the existence of some secret information which they have at their disposal, and mention decisive documents or a hidden chest whose contents they cannot divulge. In this way they can be sure that no-one will discover their secret.

Claiming decent from a royal or noble lineage is purely and simply a romantic notion. Their mother is its heroine and, but for political intrigues, their true father, a king or nobleman, would be acknowledged.

Fraud, more or less consciously executed, is a direct consequence of their condition.

Vagrancy partly stems from the miserable situations in which they find themselves, but also from their taste for adventure. Spurred on by their perpetually changing ideas, they adopt a wandering life, which represents, as it were, imagination in action. Their intellectual instability reveals itself in locomotor instability. Mrs X.'s children were drawn into this shiftless life. Sometimes those around them are not only passive instruments in this activity, but enter into the delusions themselves. The result is a *'folie à deux'* or *'délire collectif'*.

Most of these patients end up in prison. Magistrates find it difficult to accept that the mixture of lucidity and incoherence which characterises this condition is a sign of mental illness. Furthermore, the inventions are taken as evidence that the person is an impostor, an adventurer, a fraud or a blackmailer, and doctors encounter resistance from the legal profession when they argue that there is a psychiatric disorder at the root of these antisocial acts. Even if admitted to a psychiatric hospital, the patients employ their literary skill and fertile imagination to such effect, in writing letters to magistrates and appealing to public opinion, that it is difficult to insist on their detention.

Conclusion

In studying the evolution of our patient's psychosis we were struck by its persistence and how it became consolidated, partly through secondary misinterpretation but chiefly through the accumulation of further inventions and fabrications.

We believe that it represents a pathological exaggeration of a mythomanic temperament, and in this respect it resembles the misinterpretative delusional state described by Sérieux and Capgras. In this latter condition, however, it is the powers of reasoning, not imagination, which are exaggerated.

These two clinical conditions, although distinct in respect of the mechanism which gives rise to them, can be regarded as nosologically similar. In both cases, a particular mental constitution is the basis of the emergence of a profound error in mental functioning. In one case, it is an error of reasoning, and in the other a deficit in imagination. In both cases, however, the initial disorder leads to a systematised collection of delusions, without any sign of intellectual impairment.

Paul Sérieux (1864–1947)

Paul Sérieux was born in Paris. His father came from Alsace-Lorraine and his mother was English. He was attracted to psychiatry from the beginning of his medical career and was a pupil of Gaétan Magnan, one of the most influential of late 19th century French psychiatrists. He travelled widely in Germany, Italy and Switzerland and was a keen advocate of Kraepelin's ideas on dementia praecox at a time when French psychiatrists were antipathetic to them. Like other French psychiatrists whose articles are translated in this volume, he was interested in forensic psychiatry. He also wrote on the historical aspects of his subject, arguing, against established opinion, that the French Revolution had disrupted the rights of the insane and made their plight worse.

The monograph which he wrote with Joseph Capgras is a masterpiece of clinical observation combined with theoretical interpretation. The bulk of this study is translated here. More than many of the other so-called 'atypical psychoses' it deserves to be seriously considered in many cases of what are loosely termed paranoid illnesses.

Joseph Capgras (1873–1950)

Joseph Capgras was born in Central France and studied medicine in Toulouse. His cousin, who was a doctor, steered him towards psychiatry. He worked in several mental hospitals around Paris, and was then appointed to the staff of St Anne's Hospital in Paris, one of the most important psychiatric hospitals in France, where he remained until his retirement.

In addition to the present article, he is celebrated for giving a description of the syndrome which now bears his name – the Capgras Syndrome or the illusion of doubles. He was much honoured in his life-time and was an outstanding clinician and teacher.

Misinterpretative delusional states

P. Sérieux and J. Capgras (1909)

(*Les Folies Raisonnantes: le Délire d'Interprétation*, pp. 5–43. Paris: Baillière)

Introduction

A category of 'systematised delusional states', equivalent to the term 'paranoia' in other countries, has long been recognised in France. These can be acute or chronic, primary or secondary, and can occur with or without intellectual impairment. They are characterised in the main by organised groups of more or less coherent delusions relating to fantastic or absurd themes, which appear genuine to the subject. They are subdivided according to content into delusional states of persecution, grandeur, jealousy, mysticism, eroticism or hypochondria. Nowadays, however, we cannot establish the autonomy of a psychosis on the basis of delusional content alone. It is necessary to study the particular grouping of the symptoms and the full evolution of the morbid condition. As far as possible, we should try to take account of their causes and their development in the light of current psychiatric knowledge. Consequently, 'systematised delusional states' constitute no more than a morbid state which can occur at the beginning or during the course of a variety of mental illnesses.

Acute or secondary delusional states are certainly not discrete entities. The delusions are polymorphous and lack organisation; they are accompanied by excitement, depression or confusion and both their onset and termination are rapid. They may appear in the course of dementia, delirium of infective or toxic origin, certain personality disorders, affective psychosis or dementia praecox.

Chronic systematised delusional states can, however, be subdivided into two groups. The first comprises those acquired psychoses which profoundly alter the mental functions of a subject and lead sooner or later to dementia. The second group contains constitutionally determined psychoses, exaggerations of the personality which remains essentially intact. They do not lead to intellectual impairment. It is this second group which we intend to subdivide, and to identify within it a discrete nosological entity which we shall call *chronic psychosis based on delusional misinterpretation* or, in brief, *misinterpretative delusional states* by reason of their most salient feature. There are other important characteristics but, unlike the systematised psychoses which progress to dementia and originate from a disorder of perception, the states which we are considering here are almost exclusively based on delusional misinterpretation. Hallucinations, when they occur, are episodic and play almost no part in their development.

Before we outline the characteristics of this condition, we should define what we mean by delusional misinterpretation. This is a form of false reasoning, having as its point of departure a real perception, something that really happened. By virtue of its emotional associations, it then, aided by erroneous inductions or deductions, takes on an intense personal significance for the subject.

Delusional misinterpretation should be distinguished from an hallucination, which is a perception without an object, and from an illusion, which is a perception corresponding inadequately with its object. A mystic who sees the Holy Virgin appearing to him in the dark is experiencing an hallucination. Don Quixote, when he takes windmills for giants, is the victim of an illusion. We restrict the term 'illusion' to an error of the senses, although others have regarded 'misinterpretations' as 'mental illusions'. One should also beware of mistaking a misinterpretation for an hallucination; one patient, for example, claimed to have heard certain insulting words, but in the case of a misinterpretation words of some sort had actually been uttered.

Delusional misinterpretation should also be distinguished from a delusional idea, which is a false concept created out of many constituents, or at least not deduced from an observed fact. To quote Régis: 'The first is an exact point of departure, whereas the second is erroneous in its entirety; a delusional misinterpretation is to a delusional idea rather as an illusion is to an hallucination'.

It is not so easy to separate a delusional misinterpretation from a false interpretation or error. Several writers have produced useful lists of differentiating features, but none of these is entirely reliable. An error has been considered rectifiable, a delusional misinterpretation incorrigible. An error is usually isolated, circumscribed; a delusional misinterpretation tends to become diffuse and associated with analogous ideas to form a system. An error has not the self as its object; a delusional misinterpretation has, and is characterised by its markedly egocentric nature. An error does not usually have repercussions for the behaviour of a subject and often remains theoretical; a delusional misinterpretation tends to be acted on, and to orient and dominate behaviour. An error is made by a normal brain and a normal personality; a delusional misinterpretation appears on a pathological background. It is not true, moreover, that delusional misinterpretations are always recognised as absurd and unacceptable by sane people; some of them are more reasonable than many errors, and have been taken up by sensible and intelligent people.

Such affectively determined judgements are common to a variety of psychoses, and also occur in states of heightened passion; a slight emotional upset or a troublesome idea may serve to provoke them. For this reason one cannot regard the presence of delusional misinterpretations alone as a diagnostic criterion for a particular morbid entity.

We define a *misinterpretative delusional state* as: *a chronic systematised psychosis characterised by: (1) multiple and organised delusional misinterpretations; (2) the absence or infrequency of contingent hallucinations; (3) the preservation of clear consciousness and other psychological functions; (4) the progressive extension of the misinterpretations; and (5) a chronic unremitting course without a terminal dementia.* It is a functional psychosis whose origin is to be found, not in the action of a toxic agent, but in a psychopathological predisposition arising out of an anomalous development of those cerebral association areas which subserve judgement, critical sense and emotion. Essentially it is a congenital degenerative malformation.

The misinterpretative delusional state is one of the psychopathological conditions which are artificially grouped under the heading of *'folies raisonnantes'*, i.e. insanity based on faulty reasoning. Except for their 'partial delusions', subjects with this disorder retain their mental capacities and preserve their mental energy, often with remarkable skill when it comes to discussing and defending their beliefs. They hardly deserve to be called insane in the strict sense of the term because they remain in touch with their surroundings and retain the appearance of normality. Some never become psychiatric patients but only draw attention to themselves by their eccentricity. Most of them are admitted to hospital, however, not because of their ideas, but because their violent and impulsive nature renders them dangerous to other people. If one gets to know them or reads their letters or memoirs, one realises that none of their ideas is entirely unreasonable. If anything, one is struck by the logic of their opinions, the normal train of associations and the accuracy of their memory, as well as by their lively curiosity and their intact, sometimes penetrating, intelligence. One can find no evidence of active hallucinations, depression, confusion or loss of emotional responsivity. Detailed and repeated examination may be necessary to elicit the morbid ideas.

Some patients put forward quite plausible, even legitimate, complaints. A woman may accuse her husband of immoral behaviour: he has deceived her, is trying to poison her, has squandered her money and confines her to the house. A man may complain of injustice by his superiors, hostility from his colleagues and insinuations and malevolent allusions by those around him. Someone of humble birth may try to prove their connection with a titled family.

Some patients seem only to make false judgements; everything that happens is viewed from a special angle; everything is made to fit one fixed idea which is based on a false premise. Their delusional concepts remain reasonable given this first faulty step, and there is no general impairment of logical thinking.

Other patients, no different from the former in any essential respect, present their arguments in a more peculiar way. Their view of the world, although retaining an appearance of logic, becomes more and more bizarre. It soon becomes apparent that their ideas are fuelled by pathological imagination. One such patient, for example, took another inmate for a spy; nurses were police in disguise; and he soon concluded that he was surrounded by agents provocateurs in the pay of his enemies. He maintained that for a long time he had been plagued by a multitude of vexations. People were following him, whistling at him, brushing against him and spitting on him; they were making menacing gestures; they would scratch his face or touch his hands, and a woman had lifted up her skirt in front of him. During the night, doors and windows would be opened and shut to keep him awake. Various complicated obstacles were put in his path to cripple him. Why did people hang around in groups in front of a newspaper kiosk? Was it to keep him from reading certain things? He knew that newspapers were full of allusions to him, barely disguised by means of pseudonyms. His own picture appeared in the newspapers, and announcements were made about him. He was famous, he had been honoured in certain circles, a minister had taken notice of him and a woman from the nobility had looked at him with a maternal air; he must be of noble birth himself. One tries to reason with him on these matters in vain; he claims to have ample evidence to support his case.

Clinical conditions resembling our concept of misinterpretative delusional states have been noted by several French authors. Some have placed the condition along with systematised hallucinatory states, on the grounds that there is a perceptual disorder. Other psychiatrists have regarded cases with aggressive outbursts and persistent claims of injustice as representing a form of paranoia. Others have attributed clear-cut cases of what we are describing to a certain kind of personality disorder.

In our view, however, misinterpretative delusional states deserve a distinct place amongst the large group of personality disorders. They are also radically different from delusional states based on hallucinations. As for regarding them as a form of paranoia, this is an inadequate formulation because paranoia is such a heterogeneous collection of quite separate conditions . . .

In this study we shall restrict ourselves to subjects whose mental state highlights what we regard as the crucial feature of misinterpretative delusional states, namely, the pathological nature of their reasoning . . . In this way we hope to justify the autonomous position that we are claiming for these states in psychiatric classification.

Symptoms of misinterpretative delusional states

The condition is characterised by the presence of two sorts of apparently contradictory phenomena . . . On the one hand, there are positive symptoms, which owe their development to delusional misinterpretations and ideas. On the other hand, there are negative symptoms: integrity of intellectual functioning, and the absence or rare occurrence of hallucinations . . .

Delusional ideas
On cursory examination the delusional ideas appear to constitute the principal symptom, particularly the fantastic themes of their content.

Usually there are ideas of persecution or grandeur, alone, together or in sequence. Ideas of jealousy, mysticism and eroticism are frequent. Less common are hypochondriacal ideas, and occasionally there are ideas of self-accusation. The least frequent of all are ideas of possession. One never sees nihilistic ideas.

The content is of little account in understanding the nature of their delusions. What is important, and common to them all, is the way the patients defend their inventions with the help of arguments derived from reality. Although this is sometimes done in a fanciful way, most of their reasoning draws on the ordinary, the possible and the reasonable: teasing, prejudice, theft, poisoning. They never refer to supernatural powers.

The way in which these ideas coalesce into a system is very variable. It is sometimes rapid, sometimes slow; the system can be precise and incorrigible, or rudimentary and with an element of doubt; it can be poorly formulated or exceedingly complex. If the system is loosely held together, it can disturb the subject by raising numerous doubts. In some cases, it is less a question of delusional conviction than of delusional doubt; unreasonable facts are treated as possible rather than certain.

These delusional ideas are often kept secret by the patient. This is so common that one can almost regard it as a symptom. The patient so distrusts those around him that he only intimates his true thoughts by allusion and innuendo. Usually when he is first admitted to hospital he is excited and garrulous, but soon settles down to become virtually mute. This attitude poses a number of problems for the doctor. One woman kept her delusion of grandeur secret for a year, and it only emerged in her writings. A paranoid patient of Séglas and Barbé kept his delusion to himself for five years. This pattern is particularly frequent in delusions of grandeur. Sometimes these are kept hidden because the patient is aware of how unreasonable it must seem; a megalomaniac, who finally admitted that she was the sister-in-law of the King of England, added: 'I didn't talk about it because I would have been thought mad; it's so ridiculous'.

Delusional misinterpretations
Such patients do not invent what happens to them; the events are not merely figments of their imagination or fabrications of a pathological mind. The process which leads to delusions involves the distortion, dressing up and amplification of real events; the delusion is therefore more or less exclusively based on phenomena which really occurred in the outside world or in their internal world of feelings. A glance, a smile, a gesture, the cries or songs of children, a neighbour's coughing, the whispering of passers-by, a piece of paper found in the street, or an open door can all be the pretext for their misinterpretations.

The more insignificant it seems to others, the more it stands out to these patients. Where others see only coincidences, they uncover a secret truth. This ability to pick up hidden allusions, to understand insinuations and double meanings, and to interpret symbols only serves to confirm to the patient his superiority in these matters: 'I understand', he will tell us, 'things which no one else does'.

Two of Régis' patients illustrate this point very well. One said that: 'Because fate has bequeathed to me such a penetrating insight and made me always want to look beneath the surface of things I feel as if I should live alone and away from the world'. The other described how she would construct an entire sequence of events from only one fact, and how certain expressions in her conversation seemed to her as if she had guessed what she was going to say. She felt that she could predict the flow of an argument from the outset. She felt the need to offer explanations to her companions on all sorts of subjects and then interpret what followed in a certain way.

If an explanation does not spring to mind the patient will interpret this itself as significant. People, they mention, are trying to muddle them or make them lose their sense of direction. They must keep a wary eye open for such traps. Sometimes this tendency to see symbols everywhere spreads to involve their own language and behaviour. They resort to ambiguous phrases and express their thoughts in puns and riddles. A paranoid patient who had just shot someone left in front of his victim's house *'un morceau de cerceau'* [a piece of a child's hoop – untranslatable alliteration – Tr.].

Their skill in these matters appears boundless. We shall now examine the two principal ways in which misinterpretations are established, consolidated and amplified. The first we shall call *exogenous misinterpretations* – based on things which have occurred in the external world. The second – *endogenous misinterpretations* – originate from internal sensations, functional disturbances of the brain or altered states of consciousness.

Exogenous misinterpretations
Here everyday happenings are the source of most misinterpretations. A jostling in the street is a sign of impending attack. A stain on the patient's clothes is taken as a grave offence on his person. If his trousers, shoes or tie become torn or damaged this is part of a plot. If someone fails to shake their hand or does so without warmth it is an intentional slight. A dustcart passing along the street signifies malign intent. Nothing escapes their ingenuity. What do these sheets hanging out mean? Or those red curtains in the windows? Or marks on their photographs discovered after a lengthy inspection? If someone tells them about a cataract operation they are trying to suggest that they are blind to the infidelity of their partner. They are asked if the river in their home town has plenty of fish in it; this is an insinuation that they are a 'maquerau' [mackerel but also colloquially a ponce – Tr.]. Why was the son of that civil servant given the *Malade Imaginaire* to read when his father was about to take sick leave? Why do their colleagues tap their canes in that way? One woman concluded that her husband was about to leave her because she received a letter with two five centimes stamps on it instead of one of ten centimes. Another saw some shiny shoes in a shop window which he took to mean that he was a homosexual. Yet another had a special meaning for each colour: pink meant that she was

going to kill a 'baby'; white stood for her lover, Mr Blan . . . [blanc = white, Tr.] . . .

The behaviour, gestures and facial expressions of those around them play a considerable role in their misinterpretations. 'Why,' asked one patient, 'do people keep touching their eyes unless it is to tell me that I am blind? And whenever I look at the expression on Mrs A's face and particularly the way she places her finger near her nose to make a pattern as if opening a bottle of wine I wonder whose unsuspecting but nevertheless malign accomplice she is. Can it be chance or is Mrs B looking at me all the time, staring at me across the room, following my every move, and yet all the time pretending to be busy with something else?' The same patient would interpret crossed arms as meaning that her child was still alive. If people scratched their forehead it was an allusion to Mr X; if they touched their neck the gesture referred to Mr Y. The drumming of fingers on the table indicated something else. One, two or three coughs had their separate meanings, all to do with scenes from her childhood. A patient of Deny and Camus learnt by heart a book in which a particular meaning was attached to everyday objects: a needle stood for injury, an umbrella for protection, a broom for change, etc. She then made up her own symbolic language.

It is usually the most trivial incidents which lead to the most extraordinary conclusions. For example, a young woman received several glances from an actress and concluded that she was her daughter. Certain erotic delusional states are entirely based on the supposed significance of facial expression; this fact is, of course, used to good effect by playwrights and poets . . .

Sometimes the source of misinterpretations lies in important events: domestic tragedies, bereavements, unpleasant incidents. Subjects attribute the death of a parent to poisoning or to criminal activity. Some patients use national or international events as their starting point: their letters to ministers and sovereigns have decisive influence on diplomatic affairs; on their advice Russia and Japan have signed a peace treaty; their help allowed the King of England to accomplish certain missions; their money has financed several business ventures. A patient of Joffroy is interesting from this point of view. His delusional system had for a number of years been solely concerned with contemporary events: wars, catastrophes, affairs of state, sensational trials. The Dreyfus affair, the Boer War, the Russo-Japanese War, the relationship between Church and State and ministerial crises all parodied his own petty quarrels on a grand scale.

The most important symbol of all for these patients is language. They may see a personal reference in things which they hear in the street; 'Fire', 'Idiot', 'Charenton-Vincennes'. Joffroy regarded as particularly striking their habit of prefacing statements with the phrase: 'Someone told me.' Nothing annoys them more and makes them lose faith in their doctor more quickly than if they think that what they claim to have heard is taken for an hallucination.

A single innocuous phrase can give rise to the most outrageous suspicions. One patient, on being shown a portrait of a king, was told that she must surely know who it was, and concluded that it was her true father. Another heard a woman in the street saying to her child, 'Your hair looks smart', and took this to refer to his own condition . . . When out walking with his fiancée he overheard two remarks made by another couple: 'She's not for you' and 'Fashionable and enticing'. He interpreted these as comments on his engagement . . .

Sometimes the expressions that they hear take on a symbolic meaning, and they construct arguments out of the interplay and punning of these. The word 'cock' signifies pride, 'pear' an imbecile and 'rice' means that someone is laughing at them [riz = rice, rire = laugh, Tr.] . . .

Misinterpretations based on puns are often constructed from proper names. An intelligent woman believed falsely that her daughter Marie had been raped. She encountered a nurse in the hospital by the name of Marie Potin, which she took as an allusion to the rumours she had been accused of spreading about her daughter [potins – gossip, Tr.] . . .

Written material is also a potent source of misinterpretations. A particular turn of phrase, the style of the handwriting, an underlined word, spelling mistakes, punctuation or the form of the signature can all evoke suspicion. One patient told us: 'My son finished writing his name with a "u" not an "n". He has never written like that before'. Another patient thought that she recognised two styles of writing on the envelope. Another considered one of the full stops too heavy, and concluded that this negated what had been a friendly greeting.

Newspapers furnish some of the best material for such misinterpretations. Patients discover articles about themselves or messages addressed to them in the correspondence columns. There are pictures of their enemies under a false name. One patient took a picture of the King and Queen of Italy for his wife and her supposed lover . . .

Some see a complicated pattern of codes, riddles and 'interesting hieroglyphics' in newspapers or letters. They analyse, comment and translate what they see as hidden formulae. They do this in a way reminiscent of code-makers who hide certain words and leave only those which they want to form their message . . . One patient underlined the following letters in a phrase from her mother's letter: 'Tu oublies toi même' producing 'Tue-toi' [You forget yourself – kill yourself, Tr.].

Some patients go to the length of maintaining that an edition of the newspaper has been specially printed for them. 'In June 1900', wrote a patient of Legrain, 'although a regular subscriber to the newspaper Matin, I suddenly received a number of issues of this containing articles which told me quite clearly that I was the emperor of Germany. I then went to the offices of the newspaper to look up the same issues, but I could not find those articles in them. From this I concluded that an extra edition had been printed especially for me'.

Endogenous misinterpretations

(a) *Misinterpretations based on an underlying organic state.* To the numerous provoking causes emanating from the external world we also have to add *internal sensations.* The term 'somatic introspection' used by other authors is usually the expression of a misinterpretative delusional state.

A patient's deductions may arise not from any morbid trouble in his surroundings but from a detailed examination of the workings of his body. He considers certain somatic observations to be pathological simply because he has not noticed them before. Physiological phenomena, such as fatigue or an erection, serve as the point of departure of his misinterpretations. One of our paranoid subjects blamed the doctor for 'pricking feelings' and 'disordered movement' which he felt in his limbs; if, after reading his newspaper, he felt tired, this was because he was hypnotised; his wet dreams were evidence that he was being made to ingest substances without his knowledge. A woman explained her feelings of sexual arousal as the influence of some foreign and occult agent; she accused various people of having a distant effect on her genital organs.

Some patients regard poison as the cause of their condition, when it is in fact neurasthenia, tuberculosis, indigestion or colitis. During a bout of gastritis one patient believed that she had swallowed some arsenic. Another related the following experience: 'At night I am woken up by an indefinable sensation, like the rush of some fluid which relentlessly floods into my forehead, my temples and my brain; next, I feel torturing bursts of pain and buzzing in my ears. It is like molten lead or quicklime surging through my veins. It is worse after meals and in the morning, and at this time I feel as if unbelievably cruel acts are being performed'. Muscular spasms, twitches and cramps are attributed to electric currents, and insomnia, profound sleep or sleepiness after meals to drugs. During an attack of tonsillitis one patient wrote: 'I am at this moment the victim of violent changes in my throat and tonsils. Whenever I comb my hair, someone makes it all fall out. The barber scratched my face four times this morning: he is trying to make me look old; my hair is already grey like an old man; they're trying to soften my teeth to prevent me chewing properly; my blood is getting thin and I'm getting eczema as a result of all these foul things being done to me. It is only because of my personal hygiene and the strength of my constitution that I keep control of my physical and intellectual powers'.

Women may explain their menstrual problems and menopausal changes in terms of intervention by their enemies. One of our patients attributed her hot flushes to jets of fluid being played on her: 'Someone is wrinkling my skin, turning it yellow, making my cheeks hollow and pricking my eyes' . . .

(b) *Misinterpretations based on an altered mental state.* Certain altered states of consciousness and certain functional disorders can exacerbate misinterpretations. Some patients are surprised to find themselves assailed by unaccustomed thoughts or see a connection between these thoughts and events occurring at the same time. One patient was thinking of Marshal Biron, a traitor who was born in his part of the country, when at the same moment his brother walked in: he concluded that his brother had betrayed him and was his wife's lover. 'How', he then said, 'could I give an account of my whole life to my wife as if she were a confessor? It's strange. I feel as if I am being driven mad.' Another patient surprised himself by making extraordinary confessions to his parents. He felt that by such a means he was being forced to reveal his soul. Some seek, in similar ways, to understand certain feelings. If surprised to find that they have no affection for their mother, for example, they conclude that they are not a real son . . .

It is not only emotion, fatigue or nervous exhaustion which can give rise to misinterpretations. One of our patients remarked that each time he came before a magistrate he lost all his capacity for thought, would stammer and was unable to give an account of himself. He wondered what had been done to him to produce such a state. Another patient could not understand why he was so fainthearted; someone must have projected rays on to him to make him feel afraid . . .

In other cases, acute delusional states or depression supervene in the course of their condition and are interpreted as episodes of madness due to poisoning or certain suggestions.

Some patients go so far as to misinterpret previous occasions when their delusional state was particularly active.

Finally, some delusional ideas borrow their content from dreams. A patient with the mystical variety of the condition justified his preoccupation with certain themes by the nocturnal terrors he had experienced as a child. A German woman, named Katzian, had the revelation that she was not a member of the family of that name; she saw in a dream her father in prison, with a dog, a symbol of fidelity, on his right, and a cat, a symbol of faithlessness, on his left; she concluded that she was a false 'Katzian' (Katz – cat in German) . . .

Nature and formulation of the delusional ideas

Contemporary psychiatry attaches no nosological value to the nature of the delusional ideas or to the behaviour which arises from them.

The nature of delusional ideas varies, even within the same type of psychosis, according to individual factors which make up a person's psychological orientation: personality, intellectual level, inclinations, habits, education and the vicissitudes of life. All these intervene to steer the predisposed individual towards ideas of grandeur, persecution, mysticism or eroticism.

Accessory influences such as the type of schooling, cultural background, beliefs, occupation and above all social milieu also play a part. More than other psychiatric conditions, misinterpretative delusional states derive most of their content from real events – economic facts, political struggles, and scientific and industrial advances. The concerns of our patients reflect the epoch in which they live; the devils and witches which tormented paranoid subjects in the Middle Ages have given way in our day to Jesuits, Freemasons and policemen. Some people have a mentality akin to those who have lived in an earlier epoch, and they, and others who take an interest in the occult sciences, may exhibit a mixed picture of modern and medieval preoccupations.

The reactions of patients in response to their misinterpretations can also be formulated in terms of their personality . . . Apathetic and impulsive individuals may interpret an event in the same way, but react to it in opposite ways, by flight or aggression respectively. Some paranoid subjects are resigned to their fate, others fight it . . .

The predominance of a particular category of ideas gives each patient a distinctive pattern to his condition. Seven types of misinterpretative delusional states can be distinguished: persecutory, megalomanic, jealous, erotic, mystical, hypochondriacal and self-accusatory. It is exceptional to encounter any of these in a pure form, as usually two ideas become associated in the mind of a patient through either their contrasting or their similar qualities, and a crowd of further ideas produces a heterogenous collection of themes. The most frequent combination is that of grandiose and persecutory ideas. Sometimes one of the pair remains in embryonic form: for example, a persecuted individual with a streak of vanity will explain the miseries which he is undergoing in terms of the envy which brings out his grandiosity; or an ambitious person will complain of hostility from certain people. Often the two associated themes are equal in intensity and the mis-interpretations serve to satisfy fear and pride to an equal degree. The idea of jealousy is rarely found on its own; it usually derives from a sense of persecution. An erotic delution can be combined with one of jealousy and persecution. The mystical subject, usually afflicted by a special form of megalomania, often feels persecuted. The hypo-chondriacal notion is commonly episodic and has its origin in ideas about persecution. Self-accusatory ideas are ordinarily a special form of persecution . . .

Gaétan Gatian de Clérambault
(1872–1934)

de Clérambault was born in Bourges, in Central France. As a student he was attracted by artistic design, then law and finally medicine and psychiatry. His first senior psychiatric position was in a hospital for the criminally insane in Paris and he remained there for 30 years, eventually becoming its director. His two best-known contributions to psychiatric thought are his concept of mental automatism, an organic model of how certain mental functions could be split off from others; and erotomania, the false belief that one is loved, part of a wider concept of the psychoses derived from his notion of the passions.

The present extract traces his ideas on the nature of such passion-based psychoses and presents his views on erotomania, a condition which has been much discussed since.

Psychoses of passion
G. de Clérambault (1921–4)

(Les psychoses passionelles, pp. 323–7 of *Oeuvre Psychiatrique*, vol.1. Paris: Presses Universitaires de France, republished 1942)

The nature of delusional states of passion

The term *delusional states of passion* denotes all those delusional states which have as their basis a prolonged emotion, whether desire or anger. Any intense feeling can serve as the nucleus for such a state: a feeling of ownership, a sense of injustice, maternal love, religious sentiments, etc. The emotion will have been linked from the beginning with a distinct idea, and this 'ideo-affective association' then forms an indissoluble bond without affecting the general pattern of thinking. This state of affairs is not seen in misinterpretative or polymorphous states.

Autonomous states of passion exist without hallucinations, global thought disorder or dementia. There do exist, however, mixed states, where the delusional state of passion is part of some other process; we call these secondary or prodromal, depending on whether they succeed or precede the principal condition. The appearance of such 'syndromes of passion' in patients with an already abnormal mental background is explained in the following way. Patients suffering from mental disorder do not suddenly lose their affective responses, but they may at first react more intensely than normal to events. At this stage of the illness their imagination is often more active than usual, while at the same time their critical faculties are diminished. In fact, it is surprising that the freeing of the constraints on passion does not cause more problems in the course of a psychiatric illness . . . An appropriate guideline is that the intensity of experienced emotion is directly proportional to the autonomy of the condition, i.e. absence of other abnormal mental phenomena . . . For example, a normal mind has to be subjected to considerable emotion before reaching a firm conviction which goes against conventional beliefs. In this case the 'ideo-affective knot' is predominantly emotional in origin. If there is a pre-existing abnormality of psychological functioning, imaginative mechanisms become more important in the development of this 'ideo-affective knot'; a patient with general paralysis of the insane, for example, may say that he is the queen's lover, but he may not even write to her or show concern about not seeing her . . .

In addition to pure, secondary and prodromal delusional states of passion there are also the associated delusional states of passion, where two or more distinct delusions co-exist. The separate delusions are both based on strong emotions, but are different manifestations of them, for example ambition and sensitivity. Although the delusions may interact, they remain relatively independent in the way they influence behaviour . . .

Finally, there are abortive or attenuated forms of these states, where the delusion is not strongly maintained or is transient in its hold on the subject . . .

Other causes of a secondary delusional state of passion are affective psychosis and obsessional and phobic neurosis. We regard these as physiological in origin because they derive from a primitive over-arousal, unlike pure erotomania where an 'ideogenic' basis exists for the overarousal. It is not easy, however, to distinguish delusions which arise in the course of a manic-depressive or obsessional illness from those which are the central feature of delusional states of passion. Both are to some extent physiological in origin, but in the former cases the attached idea in the ideo-affective knot is unstable and easily changes to another one; in the latter case, the knot is stronger, and the idea more permanent.

Delusions secondary to a 'progressive systematic psychosis' are more easily distinguished from pure delusional states of passion. In the former case the whole range of ideas is in turmoil and other mental functions are affected. In paranoid, confabulatory and hallucinatory states, for example, it is obvious that judgement, imagination and perception, respectively, are at the root of the disorder.

Pure erotomania

The following patient is a case of pure erotomania, one of the best defined examples of a delusional state of passion.

There are no hallucinations, no generalised persecutory beliefs and no confabulatory or grandiose ideas. Erotomania is the only evidence of psychosis, the ideas are based entirely on passion and there is no progressive impairment of other mental functions. The striking features are the strength of her desire, the intensity of her reactions and the absolute conviction with which she holds her delusional beliefs. There has been no change in the content of her delusion, as one sees in polymorphous states; the belief itself is remarkably stable, and does not give way to frustration or hate. All her misinterpretations refer uniquely to the original theme and any persecutory ideas are consistent with the primary belief.

Her delusional state remained unchanged for seven years. There was no change in the object of her desire during this time and no development of persecutory, grandiose or mystical delusions.

The patient believed that a civil servant, the secretary of a government commission, was in love with her. According to her, he looked at her lovingly, sought her out, used subordinates and prostitutes to persecute her and would, sooner or later, give in to her wishes. She was aware that the man was married and did not deny that she herself had a lover whom she was about to marry. None of these facts, in her mind, constituted an obstacle to her belief.

The history dated back to 1915 when the patient needed a safe-conduct pass in order to enter the military zone. The civil servant in question had refused to give her this pass. She then plagued his office with repeated demands for the pass, and wrote seductive letters in the hope of gaining his permission. All was to no avail. She became angry and suspected that she was being unfairly treated. At one point the office lost her birth certificate and she took this as a personal affront. She resorted to extreme tactics – turning up at the office in tears, threatening suicide and writing angry letters. She was admitted to psychiatric hospitals on several occasions because of her behaviour. She was aged 34 when she first came under my care in 1919, her fifth admission in all. From our enquiries and her previous psychiatric notes, the following facts emerged. She had first been admitted to the Bicêtre asylum at the age of 12. She remained there for four years with the diagnosis of 'mental retardation, depression and suicidal tendencies'. Her mother had had a depressive illness and had committed suicide after a stillbirth. After her discharge she had become a prostitute. Then at the age of 19 she became convinced that a doctor was persecuting her. This was mainly attributable to anger, but it had an erotic component, and may have been the prelude to her eventual erotomania. She then lost contact with her relatives until the age of 33, when she had her second psychiatric admission in 1918. There were two more admissions in this year. Each time it was noted that she had persecutory ideas, that she drank heavily and that she was pursuing a civil servant whom she claimed was in love with her. She had three more admissions between then and 1922, each with the same presenting features.

The symptoms were the same in all her admissions. She had been following the civil servant and making a nuisance of herself by accosting him, attacking him and circulating scandalous stories about him. She believed that the man was in love with her, protected her in secret and, despite her conduct towards him, continued to love her . . .

The patient was misdiagnosed, in my view, by several eminent psychiatrists. Several considered that she was incapable of an independent existence but the reasons given were either her disorganisation, her impulsiveness or her alcoholism. The quarrelsome aspect to her behaviour was ignored and the erotomania went unnoticed for years.

The widespread tendency to overlook erotomania has several origins. Chief among these are the unfamiliarity of the clinical picture, and the lack of an agreed method of interviewing these patients to bring out their delusions . . .

The best interviewing technique requires a thorough acquaintance with the condition itself. An intuitive approach is of little value unless one knows what one is looking for. However, one should not proceed as if one were questioning an examination candidate. In the first place, one rarely obtains a formal declaration of the passion in question, and specific questions on this topic are either ignored or brushed aside. It is best to proceed in a more casual way, but with occasional references to the sort of ideas that one is seeking. In this way we can lead our patient gently to a state of mind in which he will feel ready to talk freely and discuss the morbid ideas, or at least feel obliged to drop hints or to pretend that he does not understand the purpose of the questions.

Either way we can gain an entry into his system of beliefs without him realising it. Patients of this kind should not, therefore, be interviewed by a series of direct questions, but rather *manoeuvred*, and in order to achieve this there is only one method – to touch on and ignite the passion in question.

The mental state of these patients is largely unrecognised in our psychiatric hospitals mainly because they do not call our attention to it by disturbing the ward, and they retain sufficient faculties to be on their guard against discovery of the real nature of their condition. Another reason why they often go unnoticed is that the psychiatrist too readily substitutes a simple banal explanation for their statements. The psychiatrist is prone to conclude falsely that 'something must have happened' to arouse their anger. Their complaints and claims of being loved are thus taken for real or slight exaggerations of reality. Another mistake is to regard their statements as consistent with a transient affective disturbance in an individual with a personality disorder . . . [De Clérambault used the traditional French term *dégeneré* for such individuals, Tr.]. Finally, the subject may be wrongly regarded as sane, responsible for his actions and therefore fit for punishment if he has contravened the law.

There are some patients whom it is difficult to distinguish in one or other of these ways. The majority, however, can easily be separated into *banal states of passion* and *morbid states of passion*. The distinguishing criteria are the *intensity of the patient's reactions*, the *persistence of their ideas* and the *incorrigibility of their beliefs*.

Secondary erotomania

The term 'secondary erotomania' is more accurate than 'associated erotomania' because it covers cases which precede (prodromal cases) as well as succeed some other condition. All such cases arise on the basis of an already disordered psychological substratum, but one can only use the term if there is already evidence of this other psychiatric condition. Prodromal erotomania is a retrospective diagnosis.

In secondary cases the erotomania is based more on imagination than on passion. It is not a sudden thing, not 'love at first sight', but a state which emerges gradually, through being worked out by the subject. There is also less energy in the pursuit of the loved one than in pure cases.

I have never seen a case of either pure or secondary erotomania in which the love was entirely platonic. In one famous case, whose love was claimed to be platonic, I discovered on interview that the patient believed she had been married to the object of her desire and had given birth to a child by him. Another case, a girl of apparently pure and impeccable virtue, was found to have sent him pictures of naked women with her own name attached.

Prodromal erotomania

Erotomania is a syndrome whose origin lies in the sphere of emotions but which has links with the faculty of imagination. In pure cases the emotional component is maximal; in secondary cases, the imaginative element predominates. Secondary cases are those where the erotomania is an integral part of a generalised psychosis.

The stability of the delusional state and the extent to which the beliefs determine action are a function of the emotional state. Thus in secondary erotomania, whether prodromal or consequential, subjects do not tend to act on their delusions, and the specific set of beliefs grows slowly and then gets reabsorbed into a protean ensemble of other abnormal beliefs and experiences. There are often changes in the object of their desire, unlike the situation in pure cases. In addition, the object may be someone whom they have never met but merely invented through imagination, misinterpretation or transformation of the content of an auditory hallucination. Sometimes the object may be determined partly by a real event in the distant past and partly by invention. We have seen this in the case of a 60-year-old woman whose erotomania centred upon someone who had been her real lover but who had disappeared from her life 30 years before. She had had a child by him, and in the intervening years had become increasingly angry with him.

All secondary cases have a substrate of a more generalised psychosis. The pre-existing psychological abnormality allows the syndrome to develop without the necessity of an emotional state. Imagination is the determining factor. In prodromal forms this psychosis remains latent, and if this is so for several years the erotomania may be mistaken for the pure type. I once saw a case like this who eventually showed signs of dementia praecox, but who for many years presented all the features of pure erotomania.

Eugene Minkowski (*c.* 1890–1972)

Eugene Minkowski was born of Jewish parents in St Petersburg, went to school in Warsaw and studied medicine in Munich. He was persuaded to take up psychiatry by his wife, who was also to become a psychiatrist, and visited Bleuler in Zurich just before the First World War. He enlisted as a volunteer in the French army in 1915 and became a battalion medical officer, serving with bravery at Verdun, the Somme and the Aisne. He was awarded the honour of 'Chevalier de la Légion d'Honneur' at the end of the war. He loved France and settled down in Paris after the war. He never had an official post in a hospital but was highly regarded as a clinician and an academic by all who knew him. During the Second World War he was persecuted because of his Jewish status.

Minkowski's importance as a writer on the theoretical aspects of schizophrenia is still underestimated. He was much influenced by the philosopher Bergson, as well as by Bleuler, and tried to combine the philosophical and the clinical approaches. The following extract is taken from his book on schizophrenia, in which he tries to understand the nature of the condition, particularly the disorder of thinking, incorporating both Bergson's and Bleuler's ideas.

The essential disorder underlying schizophrenia and schizophrenic thought

E. Minkowski (1927)

(Chapter 2, Le trouble essentiel de la schizophrénie et la pensée schizophrénique, of *La Schizophrénie*. Payot: Paris)

Vital contact with reality

In forming the concept of dementia praecox Kraepelin fused several clinical conditions which hitherto had been regarded as more or less independent. These conditions included catatonia, hebephrenia and dementia paranoides. Later the condition known as simple dementia praecox was brought in to join them.

This synthesis posed a new problem. By becoming fused, the individual symptoms and even the syndromes lost their separate value. The symptoms, according to Kraepelin, were interchangeable, inconstant and all led to the same terminal state. There must, therefore, be some shared element. They could not merely be the accidental expression of an underlying morbid process. For this reason it became necessary to reduce the richness of the symptoms and the various clinical pictures to a single fundamental disorder and to clarify its nature.

This disorder could not be sought among the ordinary clinical symptoms, such as hallucinations, delusions, catatonic manifestations or states of excitement and depression. These symptoms have nothing constant or characteristic about them as we shall see. The disorder, therefore, had to be sought on another plane. The efforts to perfect the synthesis of dementia praecox and to make a true nosological entity of it required a new look at elementary psychic functions. It is here that one hopes to find the key to the particular behaviour which all patients with dementia praecox present, despite the infinite variations which distinguish them from one another symptomatically.

Contemporary psychological notions, however, rapidly proved inadequate for this purpose. Take, for example, the traditional triad – intelligence, feeling and will. It is obvious that the disorder in question is not related to any of these faculties. Neither lack of will, indifference, inability to show emotion or, even less, intellectual deterioration are characteristic of dementia praecox. It is more a question of the selective eclipse of each of these faculties, occurring in relation to certain situations, rather than their total abolition.

Psychopathological concepts are not static. They take on new meanings as ideas about normal psychic mechanisms change. Kraepelin himself, after having talked about a weakness in the emotional impulses of will and a loss of inner unity, reduced these two disorders to a weakening of ideas and feelings, and a tendency towards a disorganised mental life. He was speaking, in this sense, of a disorder of abstraction. Under these conditions, a subject would no longer be able to transform perceptions into abstract ideas, simple feelings into more organised ones, or isolated impulses into more constant inclinations. Kraepelin even sketched out a psychophysiological hypothesis of dementia praecox, by localising this faculty of abstraction in the higher layers of the cortex. Masselon placed primary emphasis on a disorder of attention and regarded an individual with dementia praecox as being in a state of perpetual distraction. Weygandt took over Wundt's ideas and talked about apperceptive dementia. None of these concepts, based on ideas about normal psychological functioning, persisted in the long run. As they were unable to express the essential disorder of dementia praecox they eventually gave way to notions of a different type.

Expressions such as 'discordance' (Chaslin), 'intrapsychic ataxia'

(Stransky), 'intrapsychic dysharmony' (Urstein), 'loss of inner unity' (Kraepelin) or 'schizophrenia' (Bleuler) all imply that the disorder is not to be found in a particular function but rather in their total cohesion, in their harmonious interplay. To use a metaphor, the essential disorder does not affect one or more mental functions, whatever their place in the hierarchy, but is to be found among them all, in the 'interstitial space'. All these expressions constitute no more than an observation of fact, a description of the particular disturbance which occurs in dementia praecox or schizophrenia. This is already, however, an important statement, because the use of the term discordance neatly separates the condition from true dementia. But to a psychologist, and all psychiatrists should be that, this is inadequate. Chaslin's claim that hebephrenia consists of a discordance of psychic functions begs the question: what factors give rise to concordance of these same functions in normal people? This question remains for the moment unanswered. We have not yet achieved a clear idea of the fundamental disorder in dementia praecox, as we do not yet know to which factor in normal mental life it is linked.

For these reasons we have recourse to comparisons and metaphors. One might say that they suggest themselves in order to set the essentials of the condition in relief. Kraepelin talked of an 'orchestra without a conductor' and Chaslin of a 'machine without fuel' which, because it could be set in motion again, was entirely different from a broken-down machine. Anglade disliked using the term dementia praecox; he talked simply of 'dissociated patients'. To characterise their state, he compared them to a second-hand book: the pages might be out of place and the text partly illegible but none of the pages was actually missing. Compare this with a book whose pages have been irretrievably torn out. I myself, in thinking of the schizophrenic process, have been attracted by the following image: a building is made of bricks and cement; either the bricks *or* the cement can crumble; in either case the whole edifice can no longer hold up and it collapses; however, the ruins are not the same; they look different and have a different value; it is, moreover, easier to reconstruct a new house with intact bricks than with dust.

These metaphors express as well as possible the need to separate the schizophrenic process from intellectual impairment. But more than this, they seem to express the true nature of schizophrenia much better than any of the psychological definitions which we considered above.

Our sense of precision, however, is upset by these metaphors, which seem to be merely ingenious and pleasant methods of discourse.

Scientific method and the search for truth should forbid such diversions. However, one should not forget that Henri Bergson, one of the most eminent of contemporary philosophers, believes that a whole side of our life, and not the least important, entirely escapes discursive thought. Things which impinge immediately on our consciousness, in some ways the most essential, belong to this category. They are irrational but are no less part of our life for that. There is no reason to sacrifice them to the spirit of precision. In fact, on the contrary, one should try and capture their true essence. The discipline of psychology has nothing to say on this matter as it is too constrained by the rules of scientific method. Were it to relax these rules it would be transformed from an arid subject to a fertile one, and would come to resemble life itself. How would we profit from this transformation in tackling the problem of schizophrenia?

It is at this point that the idea emerges of *vital contact with reality.*

Bleuler laid down what he saw as the cardinal symptoms of schizophrenia. They were all to do with the ideas, emotions and will of his patients. At the same time, however, his introduction of the concept of autism rendered environmental factors increasingly important. His emphasis on the lack of real goals and guiding ideas, and absence of emotional warmth, steered the concept of schizophrenia down a new path. All these disorders seem to converge on a single and unique notion, that of *loss of vital contact with reality.*

Vital contact with reality appears to be linked with the irrational factors in life. The ordinary concepts elaborated by physiology and psychology, such as excitation, sensation, reflexes and motor reactions, continue in parallel, largely unnoticed. The blind, the mutilated and the paralysed may be able to live in even more intimate contact with their environment than individuals whose sight is intact and whose limbs are whole; schizophrenics, on the other hand, can lose this contact even with an intact sensory-motor apparatus, memory or intelligence. The vital contact with reality is in touch with the depths, with the very essence of our personality, in which it links with the world around us. And this world is not just a collection of external stimuli, of atoms, forces and energy. It is a moving stream which envelops us at all points and constitutes the milieu without which we would not know how to live. 'Events' emerge from this like islets; they penetrate the personality by disturbing its most intimate parts. And then, by making these events part of its own make-up, our personality puts its own stamp on them, not by muscular contractions but through action, feelings, joy and tears. In this way there is established that marvellous harmony between ourselves and reality, a harmony that allows us to follow the progress of the world while at the same time safeguarding the notion of our own life.

These considerations lead one to conclude that vital contact with reality concerns the intimate dynamism of our life. We can never achieve this through the rigid concepts of spatial thought. Metaphors, not definitions, hold pride of place in this sphere of our life. Only they can impart some clarity to the notion of vital contact with reality.

This notion is not new. In his theory of psychasthenia Janet talks at length about the reality function. This idea, although not quite the same as ours, has many points in common with it. And the fact that two different paths lead in the same direction suggests that we are dealing with real and important matters which are currently 'in the air'.

The notion of a vital contact with reality, and the interpretation of schizophrenia in terms of a loss of this contact, is both simple and plausible. The newcomer to psychiatry can pick it up quickly and use it without difficulty. I am tempted to say that the notion follows on naturally from the evolution of the concept of dementia praecox.

But then, one might ask, has the considerable knowledge about clinical psychiatry merely led, in the end, to no more than a single psychological and psychopathological idea? I do not think so. As we shall see, the idea is capable of fostering further developments, and even if this were not so it is of some consequence in its own right, as is the case with many other clinical notions in psychiatry. The term 'mental confusion', for example, owes its origin to the need to tighten up the boundaries of dementia. It replaced the category of acute, curable dementia introduced by Pinel. Originally a French idea, promoted by Delasiauve, it was then exported to other countries. In the course of its evolution, having undergone many alterations in meaning, it is again being studied in its country of origin, particularly by Chaslin. Finally, through the efforts of Toulouse and Mignard, it has come to mean a general disorder of mental functions. This pattern in the evolution of our clinical notions in psychiatry should not surprise us. Does not any clinical term become clear and precise when we have succeeded in giving it a solid psychological foundation? Also we should appreciate that modern psychiatry strives to uncover the *causative disorder* underlying the clinical conditions which it studies.

I believe that I have staked a claim for the correct paternity of the idea of vital contact with reality in respect of its central role in schizophrenia. I have certainly not invented it, for ideas which have no link with past or present are usually of little value. On the one hand, the work of Bergson has influenced me greatly. On the other hand, Bleuler's book on schizophrenia contains the notion of a profound disturbance in the relationship with the outside world. Bleuler, however, laid most emphasis on the cardinal and elementary symptoms in this condition, symptoms which arise through the attrition of the ideas, emotions and will of the patient. Although he mentioned loss of contact with reality (autism), he did not regard this as the cause of these symptoms. A vital contact with reality, in his view, was not an essential regulatory factor in life to which other mental functions were subordinate. Faithful to associationism, he put forward, in his theory of schizophrenia, the opinion that a particular disorder in the association of ideas was at the root of this condition. He then looked for an underlying organic substrate.

In introducing French psychiatrists to the notion of schizophrenia, I cannot avoid a personal note. When one has genuinely tried to understand someone else's ideas, to live them rather than merely to adopt them, it is not always possible to be dispassionate. But this is of little significance. Science advances through the efforts of its practitioners, but we are merely agents and not part of the actual process.

In putting forward the idea that a vital contact with reality is central to the understanding of schizophrenia, I am aware that there is a certain conflict between Bleuler's work and my own analysis. The difference is well set out by Villey-Desmésaret, and the French psychiatrist Claude supports my point of view: 'We are struck by the fact that the profound disequilibrium in the contact with reality is not just a consequence of some other mental disorder, but is itself the underlying disturbance out of which emerge all the cardinal symptoms of this condition'.

The notion of a loss of vital contact with reality as the essential disorder in schizophrenia has led me to consider how this deficit could be formulated further. I shall try to present the evidence in the following pages.

Intellectual dementia and schizophrenic dementia

It is now necessary to look at the consequences of the disorder which we have just outlined. Bergson, in particular, has influenced my thinking on these matters. As we saw in the previous section, my notion of vital conduct with reality is itself a point of contact between the Zurich school of psychiatry and Bergsonian ideas. I also believe that psychology and psychopathology benefit from having closer links with philosophy.

It is hardly necessary to set out Bergson's ideas in detail. The main thing to remember is his maxim that intelligence and instinct are in fundamental conflict. 'Instinct', says Bergson, 'is modelled along the same lines as life itself; intelligence, on the other hand, is characterised by a complete lack of understanding of life'.

Intelligence, although it is the product of nature, has as its principal object inorganic matter. It can only reflect things which are discontinuous and immobile. It only feels at home when dealing with dead things. It always acts as if it were fascinated by the contemplation of inert matter. Hence it is disturbed when faced with living things and finds itself face to face with organisation.

From the very fact that it is always striving to reconstruct what is there, intelligence cannot capture what is new at any moment in history. It has no room for the unpredictable. It rejects anything creative. Preoccupied only by repetition and similarity, intelligence cannot appreciate the changes produced by time. It ignores the fluidity inherent in things, and petrifies everything it touches. 'We may not think in real time, but we live in it' (Bergson).

Psychopathology cannot be expected to provide a complete answer as to whether Bergson's ideas shed any new light on problems which current psychological thinking has by-passed. They may do so, however, because morbid processes, by acting selectively, can 'dissect' the various psychological functions and reveal them in their naked state. Pathology sometimes succeeds where physiological methods fail to unravel the complexity of the factors involved.

Intelligence and instinct, i.e. the part of our mind dealing with solid inert and spatial aspects of reality on the one hand, and the part dealing with temporal and dynamic considerations on the other hand, are normally fused harmoniously. On its own neither can account for existence, but together they are complementary while at the same time limiting the other's sphere of influence in an entirely natural and appropriate way. But can this harmony be undermined by pathogenic influences? Cannot instinct, for example, be damaged on its own? Would not intelligence, in such circumstances, freed from its natural restraints, try to make up for the missing instinct and come up with bizarre ideas? Conversely, could not intelligence be the seat of a primary lesion with secondary involvement of other factors, depending on its chronicity? Questions of this type do not lead to abstract speculations. On the contrary, they lead, as we shall see shortly, to a series of facts which have been neglected by earlier investigators of psychopathology.

First, let us compare, in this respect, the two major mental processes which psychopathology has so far separated – schizophrenia and intellectual impairment. Most writers in recent times have insisted on a fundamental difference between these two. Nonetheless, it is not easy to say precisely in what this difference consists. We can say with some certainty that intellectual impairment affects judgement and memory. But there is no such certainty about the schizophrenic deficit. The term 'dementia' provides a very poor description of its essential nature.

To quote Bleuler: 'In schizophrenia, even when well-advanced, all the simple mental functions, as far as we know, are intact. In particular, memory, unlike the case in true dementia, is unaffected . . . One may find surprisingly that under an apparent envelope of dementia the intelligence is much less affected than one might imagine, as if it were only asleep'. Or, as Chaslin noted: 'It is as if in discordant insanity (schizophrenia) the symptoms resemble those of true dementia. The cold delirious incoherence, the indifference, the bizarre acts, the complete cessation of intellectual activity and its substitution by behaviour of an inferior order, the stupor and bizarre postures, and the incoherent actions all suggest this. Despite the symptomatology, however, there is rarely any sign of true intellectual impairment, such as loss of memory or errors of judgement . . . In contrast to genuine organic dementia, where the intellectual functioning is actually worse than it appears at first sight, in the discordant form of insanity nothing seems to have been irretrievably lost and only a little effort seems to be required to revive the cerebral activity'.

What, then, is lacking in schizophrenia? And what is the key to the difference between it and true dementia? It is this very difference which we will try to uncover by making use of the opposition of intelligence and instinct which we discussed earlier. As well as noting the differences in psychological *deficits* between these two conditions we shall also draw attention to differences in *intact functioning* between them.

We will begin the study of the two processes by comparing the extreme degrees of deterioration which can occur in each.

We have chosen general paralysis of the insane as a good example of intellectual impairment. For our purpose this condition has the advantage that it usually affects individuals in the prime of life. The intellectual impairment is not then complicated by other factors, such as the physiological consequences of old age, which affects senile dementia. It exists, therefore, in a relatively pure state.

If I ask someone with general paralysis: 'Where are you?' he will reply: 'Here.' Lest he is only responding in a purely verbal and automatic way, I insist: 'But where is here?' The patient taps his foot to indicate the place where he is, or points to it with his finger, or even demonstrates the room with a gesture. 'But here', he says to us, apparently surprised and annoyed by our insistence on the matter.

There is no question here of some simple semi-automatic response. This type of reply is found surprisingly often in these patients.

The schizophrenic, on the other hand, in reply to the same question, will give the name of the place quite correctly. But he will often say that, although he *knows* where he is, he does not *feel* as if he is in that place, or that he does not feel as if he is in his body. The term 'I exist' has no real meaning for him.

Two different types of factor are involved in our spatial orientation. There are those static factors concerned with the appreciation of how objects relate to one another in a geometrical space where everything is immobile, relative and reversible. But in fact we *live* in space, and we are always aware of the notion: 'I am here at this instant'. Under normal circumstances, therefore, our spatial concepts must accommodate this awareness. Our knowledge of things and our memory images come to be grouped around the notion of 'I am here at this instant'. This allows us to tell in any set of conditions where we are: in Paris, for example, or in Finland, or at our desk.

In patients with general paralysis, the static factors that I discussed earlier, the knowledge of things and memory, are impaired. Such patients are disorientated in space, in the usual sense of the word. Despite this, the structure of their notion of themselves as being 'me in this place' remains intact and active. Schizophrenics, by contrast, know where they are, but their notion of 'me in this place' has no longer its usual quality and finally breaks down.

At a less advanced stage of general paralysis we encounter reactions which are more complex, but whose general character is the same. To the question: 'Where do you come from?' the patient will reply: 'From over there, where I was before'. He is clearly disorientated in space, and unable to name the place where he came from. Nonetheless, the internal representation of a change in place – place X before and place Y now – remains intact.

The following statements belong to the same category:

Q. 'Where are you?'	A. 'Here where I was washing myself this morning' or 'Here where I have been for some time now'.
Q. 'What is this building?'	A. 'It is the building where I have been put'.
Q. 'Who is this gentleman?'	A. 'He is someone who is here'.
Q. 'What are you doing?'	A. 'At the moment I am staying here'.

If we put someone with general paralysis in front of a mirror and ask: 'Whom can you see in there?' he will reply: 'Me'. But if we continue: 'But who is me?' he will not give his name or his job. This sort of reply is much less common in schizophrenics, even in states of deterioration. They will reply: 'Me' and then 'my activity, my personality', or 'It is energy', or, abandoning their delusions, simply state 'Me, the son of Claude Farrère'. One of our patients replied: 'I know who it is' but then admitted that she no longer experienced it in the same way: 'I know who it is, but this is merely an observation, there is nothing inside; it's a queer face; it has a fixed look, oblique and cold'.

The patient with general paralysis, even in the final stages of mental deterioration, retains some sense of awareness of self. The schizophrenic, on the other hand, does not, and is always affected by a sense of depersonalisation.

A sort of commonsense and a knowledge of where to find things is also retained in general paralysis. One such patient, when asked the date, picked up a newspaper. Another very demented patient on being asked 'What day is it?' replied: 'I have no means of knowing'. Another, asked to give his date of birth, replied: 'I can't say; I haven't got my wedding ring'. On his wedding ring he would not find his date of birth but the date of his marriage [French tradition, Tr.] but that is not the point; he knew that there are ways of compensating for a failing memory and instinctively used them.

The behaviour of a schizophrenic is quite different. He usually knows the date, but the knowledge has no precise meaning for him; he cannot use it in a fashion appropriate to his circumstances. The *pragmatic* use of things is affected early in this condition.

A patient with general paralysis, in a state of profound dementia, was asked: 'What are you doing?' He replied: 'I am waiting for something to happen and making plans'. Another patient, although so deteriorated that he could no longer speak, still noticed that I had left my hat in his room one day and laughed about it. For the schizophrenic such events or manoeuvres would pass him by.

These various comparisons establish what is a fundamental difference between the intellectual impairment in general paralysis and schizophrenic deterioration. We must not confuse them. In the former case the deficit is in static mental functions; in the latter dynamic factors bear the brunt of the morbid process.

This formula is obviously too schematic. The word 'dynamism' for instance is ambiguous. It can be given a physical interpretation. But here, as in the study of movement, as Bergson pointed out, time is already conceived as a straight line and assimilated within a spatial context.

True dynamism, as it relates to our actual experience of time, is entirely different. We can only glimpse its real nature in an imperfect and provisional way. A solid base for our ideas about it does not exist. To make some advance in knowledge we can only describe and group the phenomena in our life which have a bearing on real time and then see how they fit together in both normal and morbid states of mind. In this way we can begin to construct a psychology and a psychopathology of time as we experience it. This is undoubtedly a difficult task, but one which is indispensable for anyone who wants to understand the normal and pathological functioning of the human mind.

While awaiting further studies on these matters, I believe that my own formula provides a reasonable summary of current knowledge . . . Let us examine general paralysis in more detail. In early cases the characteristics which I have just outlined are attenuated but can still be discerned. The appreciation of the passing of years, months or weeks, i.e. the notion of measurable duration linked to spatial events, is often lost, but this does not mean that such patients lose all sense of time. They may be able to give a correct account in chronological order of what they did during the war, but are no longer able to say when the war started or finished. Their memory for a succession of discrete events is preserved but their ability to relate this to a fixed point in time seems to be lost.

Spatial images to do with the passage of time also disappear. In their place, certain elements of the notion of time, now freed from the constraints of these spatial images, become more prominent and pervade the entire psychological apparatus. All the crazy ideas and plans of such patients have the quality of immediacy and have to be carried out quickly. Expressions such as 'soon', 'immediately', 'not long ago' and 'shortly' appear with surprising frequency in the things they say. One patient was always talking about how her husband, according to her, had to come and find her. She believed that he was already there, climbing the stairs or actually in her room. Or patients may talk about cars speeding at 500 miles an hour, or journeys they have made to Argentina which lasted only five minutes.

This dynamism invades the entire being of the patients, overwhelms them and appears to open up the entire universe to their stream of thought. These, then, are the symptoms of the delirious phase of general paralysis. The patient makes plans for the immediate future, grandiose schemes with no limits. He aims to go straight away to the racecourse and then make a world trip. He will blow up all the islands in the world and then collect the moon to put in a glass. He is all-powerful, feeling that he can do whatever he likes: undertake organ transplants, engage in cross-breeding animals, bring the dead back to life. He extends his extraordinary powers to all living things. He distributes his millions, wants everyone to be happy and invites all the doctors and nurses on his fantastic voyages. He is going to go to Rome to demand that all priests and nuns should be allowed to marry; he wants to set free all the fish in the world.

Everything has to do with movement here. There is nothing but vast, rapid movement. No obstacle is considered, no distance is too great and no time limits are set. The patient interprets this state of affairs in everyday language, with the help of ideas which everyone knows are absurdly grandiose.

Let us now compare this picture with the way a schizophrenic, after several years of illness, depicts his state of mind:

> Everything seems immobile around me. Things present themselves in isolation, on their own, without evoking any response in me. Some things which ought to bring back a memory, or conjure up a thought or give rise to a picture, remain isolated. They seem to be understood rather than experienced. It is as if a pantomime were going on around me, one which I cannot take part in. There is nothing wrong with my judgement but I seem to lack any instinctive feel for life. I don't seem to be able to act with any vigour. I can't change from one emotion to another and how can you live like that. I've lost contact with all sorts of things. The value and complexity of things no longer exists. There's no link between them and me. I can't immerse and forget myself in a task anymore. There's a barrier all round me. I've even less flexibility when I think about the future than I have about the present and the past. There's a kind of routine affecting me which does not allow me to contemplate the future. The creative ability in me has gone. I see the future only as a repetition of the past.

This account is taken from a patient who spent all her days in bed in a state of complete inertia and who, when she got up, behaved like an automaton. She had auditory hallucinations and delusions of bodily change, and on one occasion had set fire to her clothes in order, as she explained, to experience real sensations which were totally lacking under normal circumstances.

Do not such statements give a clue to the disorder underlying schizophrenia? They are so common in the histories of schizophrenics that we cannot avoid giving some weight to them. Time and again we hear them say: 'My ideas are immobile like a statue' or 'I feel static and lack a sense of reality'. These and other similar expressions reflect the fact that they are gradually being taken over by a sense of immobility, which, if they are aware of it, they find very unpleasant. Their posture and behaviour bear the stamp of this morbid immobility. It shows itself in their stereotyped movements, which are a kind of perpetual repetition of one movement.

It is hard to imagine a more extreme contrast between this clinical picture and that of general paralysis described earlier.

This contrast is also stressed by other writers on the matter. Kraepelin, for example, gave the specific nature of the terminal state an important role in his notion of dementia praecox. He talked in this case of '*Verblödung*'. Nayrac, discussing the meaning of this term, wrote:

> Most writers have translated this word as dementia, but this has led to much confusion. In my view the word *Verblödung* means something different. I do not say this because of a desire to be pedantic. I genuinely think another word is needed. *Verblödung* denotes making someone feel shy and ashamed to such a degree that they look intellectually backward. For want of an equivalent expression in French, we have translated *Verblödung* as 'paradementia'.

Bleuler talked about *affective dementia* in schizophrenia, emphasising yet again the fundamental difference between the deterioration in schizophrenia and the intellectual decline in dementia. I myself am more concerned with factors underlying the disintegration of the personality, and I prefer to talk about *pragmatic dementia*. The juxta-position of these two terms (pragmatic and dementia) is not altogether fortunate. I think that it would be better to omit the word dementia altogether, if this expression denotes a progressive decline in intellectual functions, and to talk instead of a *pragmatic deficit*. Whatever one thinks of this proposed term, it seems to hit on some grain of truth about schizophrenia. Claude and his pupils came to a similar conclusion in their study of schizomania, suggesting that in these cases there was an incongruity between intellectual and pragmatic activity.

Finally, I should like to draw attention to the definition of dementia praecox put forward by Dide and Guiraud:

> The condition is characterised by the sudden weakening, at an early age, of the instinctual drives of mental life, stemming directly from organic brain damage. Purely intellectual operations are only affected secondarily; they do not disappear, but are obstructed and made to work in a contradictory manner. The decline in vital spirit and strength of emotions is the necessary and sufficient element by which we can characterise the illness.

Dide and Guiraud suggested the term 'juvenile athymhormia' as a replacement for dementia praecox.

Putting on one side the organic interpretation of Dide and Guiraud, I agree with their ideas on the psychological nature of schizophrenia. They also confirm what Kraepelin and Bleuler have taught for some time, namely that dementia praecox is not a true dementia because spontaneous cures, impossible to predict, may occur years after the onset of the illness, in subjects who have had all the external signs of a complete and permanent deterioration.

Spatial thought in schizophrenia (morbid rationalisation and morbid preoccupation with geometry)

This is not the place to review all the psychopathological consequences of the primary disorder discussed earlier. I shall restrict myself to one or two examples, and indicate the direction in which I think psychological research should go. We shall see that schizophrenics, deprived of the ability to assimilate those aspects of reality which have to do with movement or time, tend to rely on the logical and mathematical side of experience. Life itself cannot be reduced to these latter factors, and any attempt to do so can only lead to a distorted view of it.

Consider the following case history which I have published under the title 'morbid rationalisation'.

The patient was a teacher, aged 32, who was referred to us at the Clinic for the Prevention of Mental Disorders. He complained at first of a 'physiological decomposition' which was causing him discomfort, and an 'emptiness in the head' which he attributed to excessive salivation. His voice, he maintained, was influencing him in a suggestive way; it seemed 'dead' and seemed to be a 'ghost voice'. His whole being had undergone 'a regression', and he felt as if he were again 15 years old, when he was a young student.

The patient had neither hallucinations nor delusions. There was no sign of intellectual decline, but from the first interview we were struck by his behaviour. This impression grew stronger in the course of subsequent interviews. His profoundly morbid attitude led to a diagnosis of schizophrenia, of a severe and well advanced form.

It is this attitude that I shall now try to describe as well as possible. The following incident was very characteristic. The patient told us that for several years now he had been interested in philosophical problems. He had been in the habit of writing down his thoughts and had amassed a considerable stack of notes. We asked him if he had read many philosophical works. He replied: 'No, on the contrary, I purposely avoided them so as not to spoil my own thoughts'. He shunned the company of other people, 'so as not to be disturbed in my reflections'. His morbid attitude is here shown in its clearest form. He was isolating himself from the world in order to keep within himself the source of his philosophical thoughts. We were not at all surprised to find that one of his theories concerned 'the way acid acting on nerve terminals gives rise to human behaviour'.

This strange attitude cannot be regarded as a disorder of judgement because then it would be necessary to ask why it takes this form rather than any other. In my view it has more to do with the morbid attitude which I have been discussing in this paper.

All of us need from time to time to withdraw from our surroundings and to commune with ourselves. In this way we draw strength to continue our mental activity and work. But we do not then totally reject all outside influence on our personality. On the contrary we allow our environment to interact with ourselves and recast our inner life according to the elements of this environment which affect us deeply. At the same time we do not allow our surroundings to dictate our entire life because we would then be enslaved by it. There must be some mechanism in normal people whereby the influence of one's environment and one's originality are kept in balance. It seems to me that this is an essential part of the human condition, and one which is difficult to describe in logical terms. We might designate it as a *feeling of harmony with life*.

It is essentially irrational, in the sense that our intellect cannot comprehend it completely, but this feeling enters into all the important situations which we encounter and is the source of most of our conflicts. Moreover, it is the basis for most of our decisions about the way we live because it gives *limits and strength* to these decisions which our intellect alone cannot provide.

Every major decision is determined by this feeling of *harmony with life* but, because the latter is not open to our scrutiny, its precise influence can never be quantified, and the decisions themselves may, therefore, appear irrational. As Pascal said: 'The heart has its reasons which pure reasoning can never uncover'. I am tempted to alter this to: 'Life has its reasons which pure reasoning cannot formulate'.

Returning to our patient's strange attitude, we can describe his psychological state in the following way. His mental energy, instead of being directed towards an integration with reality, entirely ignores the real world around him, and without any natural anchor for it to function the patient loses himself in the clouds. Not being a philosopher, even a second-rate one, our teacher ties himself up in knots with his own philosophical speculations. At the same time he rationalises his feeling of isolation by developing the notion that he does not want to be disturbed in his thoughts, and by doing so he cuts himself off from human contact.

The richness and variety of life disappears in the course of this process. However powerful an intellect may be, it cannot be entirely self-sufficient. Thinking and acting without taking into account the ideas of others or external circumstances is bound to lead to errors and absurdities.

We have analysed in some detail a single statement of this patient – i.e. 'I do not want to be disturbed in my thoughts' – because it seems to contain a distillation of his whole way of being and his relationship with the outside world.

Any act that we carry out can be regarded as an antithesis between yes and no, between good and bad, between what is allowed and what is forbidden, or between what is useful and what is harmful. We can talk in this sense of an antithetical attitude. It is the result of a lack of the irrational feeling of harmony with oneself and life, which we mentioned earlier, and indicates a total loss of ideas about the limits and strength of our intellectual activity. A person who follows this course will only behave in accordance with his own ideas and will become as a result doctrinaire and pedantic. It may be an advantage when it comes to solving mathematical problems, but it is morbid and dangerous when we are faced with practical issues and need guidance in our actions and our decisions. An example should make this clear. Our patient said that he 'always examined actions with a fine tooth comb' to see if they were in accord with his principles. His desire to be spiritually perfect led him to 'banish from existence all material work'. Before his illness he would devote all his leisure time to bee-keeping, but then, because he regarded it as material work, he completely neglected it. Whenever his parents, with whom he lived, brought up the question of money, he would see this as an attack on his ideals and avoid the conversation. He regarded his visit to the clinic as 'moral suicide', because he believed that 'man should be self-sufficient and should be under no other authority'. This is in itself logical, but is here taken to extreme lengths. His comment shows that principles can have absurd consequences by reason of inappropriate generalisation. Life is not made up of rigid and universal principles; there is always a built-in measure of irrationality which determines the limits of reason.

The patient's moral regeneration, he stated, began in 1918 while he was in a prisoner-of-war camp in Germany. He tried at that time to detach himself from material things and be directed in his behaviour by impersonal principles. He thought it right to achieve wisdom as the only true form of happiness, but for this purpose he had to be alone, removed from any disturbing elements. Under the influence of these ideas his personality was transformed. He devised a set of rules by which to live. These included temperance, silence, and the application of a new principle every week. He virtually ceased talking and would only answer questions when these were in conformity with his principles. His actions were regulated minute by minute. He believed that his problems only began when he allowed himself, against his principles, to talk impulsively. After the war he returned to his job as a teacher. At first he tried to apply to his teaching the principle of absolute indulgence, because he believed that his pupils were irresponsible. They laughed at him and had no idea what he was getting at. Next, at the suggestion of his headmaster, he applied a strict military regime. Then there followed a period of 'liberalism and gentleness'. He wrote in his diaries at this time:

> I put into practice, until last June, an impersonal discipline, firm and confident in my mind that I was encouraging a dignity in behaviour and thoughts. Inspired by logic, I had to stifle my idealist tendencies for a whole year in order to maintain military discipline. I carried out one or two manual tasks to please my parents, but this subordination of my actions to the wishes of two old people made me even more vulnerable to their sentimental assaults, which hitherto I had been able to withstand by my powerful humanitarian feelings. I soon found myself an obedient child. Any attempt at initiative seemed futile and I felt suffocated.

This, in brief, was the patient's attitude. In keeping with his antithetical outlook, he saw any outside force as an attack on his personality; if he succumbed to it he would be dragged down and engulfed. He could only register outside influences as having a hold on him or as a trap.

How different he is in this respect from normal people! The bonds which attach us to our environment are infinitely more rich and complex. We may try to impose our will on others and dominate our immediate social circle; at the same time we know how to do our duty, to respond to love or pity, to recognise the authority of others and to follow their advice, without feeling any constraint on our freedom. Our teacher recognised only two categories: independence, which through his egocentricity he only achieved at opposite poles of his intellectual antithesis; and domination, which he continually suffered. He would only admit to being ill for two months, although in our view it had been much longer. He attributed the onset of his illness to his succumbing to suggestions from his parents which had affected his voice and made him emit ideas which went against his principles. He felt that he had lost control over himself and that he was behaving as if he were carrying out orders from another person. Whereas before he had felt master of the way he looked or talked, now, when teaching in class, he felt in the sway of the sound of his own voice, and his gaze would fix, against his wishes, on the pupils. He had lost his desire to teach because he felt that his work and principles were being directly controlled by the headmaster.

It is unlikely that the way in which the teacher behaved was really a result of a conscious effort on his part, as he would have had us believe. It is more probable, as discussed earlier, that a regulatory factor in his life was missing and that the remaining elements regrouped to form some unifying whole. The patient then interpreted this intellectually as a coherent system, but it was in fact distorting his whole action and turning him into a 'stranger', we might almost say an 'alien', in his relationship with his environment and ourselves.

I should also like to comment on the way in which the world around him affected the patient's altered mental state. In this respect, his lack of vital contact with his environment and the disharmony of his mind are the main factors.

The patient's state of consciousness may be compared to that of a stage on which abstract principles enter and compete for attention. It was altogether a very impersonal stage, and he must have treated these principles accordingly. We saw that his pupils took no notice of his doctrines, probably because there was no warmth, no intimacy and no personal touch in the way he applied them. He had lost, one might say, the sensitivity which allows us to communicate with others, to feel with them and to enter into their concerns. The ability to make personal rapport was shattered and he no longer knew even how to look at people in a natural way. His sphere of interest might seem much wider than is usual, indeed almost boundless, but this is an artefact of the despair of a spirit deprived of affinity with normal concerns. He would tell us that he had become 'detached from material things and was only governed by impersonal principles', and that he was no longer under the influence of a *restraining milieu* but of the *entire* world. He lived for ideas and saw people as impersonal objects. He was kept going by thoughts, not people. He could appreciate a sense of humanity but always sought to achieve the absolute in this regard. His filial love was drowned by a much grander love. It is not surprising therefore, for someone who saw things in this way, that minor arguments between him and his parents became in his mind a veritable battle of giants. His parents, concerned at his bizarre attitude, tried to intervene. His father pointed out that if you cannot carry a load of 100 kilos on your back, you should try 50 kilos. In response to this and other such statements involving material topics, our patient only became more convinced that his ideals were under attack. His belief that his parents were trying to undermine his personality became stronger, and if he tried to make the slightest concession he immediately felt he was renouncing his ideals on a massive scale.

When recounting the story of his life he would merely give a list of the ideas and principles which he had adopted, as in the account of his teaching career – the periods of indulgence, of military discipline, and of liberalism. His whole life seemed to have evolved in fits and starts. It was not a continuous line, supple and elastic, but one that was broken in several places. The ideas which he had entertained seemed also to have appeared in isolation, with no links between them. This had also been the case with the rules governing his life, which were self-contradictory or incompatible with each other. Emotional factors and, even more striking, the sense of time seemed to have entirely disappeared from our teacher's existence. He was also continually in 'conflict with life'.

Let us compare this man with another patient who said that he could not be sure of the importance of money, because money did not take up much space. This patient had also said that he did not find change very interesting because everywhere he went he was always finding 'too much change, too much mobility'. Instead, his attention was completely absorbed in a project to enlarge the Gare de l'Est in Paris, which was in all the newspapers at the time. He invested it with enormous importance, exceeding all other events in his life.

In this case there seemed to be an abnormal generalisation concerning ideas about spatial order which had a morbid hold on his thinking and behaviour. This involved the application of mathematical criteria to determine the value of objects and events solely in terms of their dimensions or geometrical characteristics.

Do we not see here the first signs of what might be called a *morbid preoccupation with geometry*?

The same patient revealed that from the age of 16 he had been 'obsessed', as he put it, by the subject of construction. He would doubt the solidity of things and wondered if the walls of his school were straight.

> 'I was tormented,' he wrote in his autobiography, 'by the vaults in churches. I could not accept that all that weight could be supported by ribs, pillars and a keystone. I could not understand way it did not fall down. I could not see why the cement in the free stones did not crumble because it must be a particularly vulnerable pressure point. I concluded that houses stayed up only through some terrestrial attraction. I came to doubt my own senses.'

A 'mania for symmetry' then took hold of him, and also an 'obsession with pockets'. He wanted to know what difference there was between putting one's hands straight into a normal jacket pocket and putting them into the sloping pockets of an overcoat. He solved this problem by concluding that 'in the first instance you establish a feeling of parallelism between extreme things, arms and legs'.

He also had the habit of standing in front of a mirror, legs together, trying to place his body symmetrically, to achieve, as he said, 'an absolutely perfect position'. To this end, he would hold his breath as long as he could.

During his military service he had once been given an injection. The idea had then grown on him that a piece of cottonwool had entered his body along with the injected fluid. He then constructed a vast series of ramifications from this single idea, all following a geometrical and rational pattern:

> The obsession grew and grew. It was no longer just cottonwool that had been inserted, it was the metal from the needle as well, the glass from the syringe; each organ in my body was systematically affected, until my brain was involved. I thought the substance which they had injected was poisonous, and so were all the injections I had had afterwards. And I also drew things which had happened before that into my obsession. Any treatment was useless. I had to uncover the cause of it all right down to its roots, right down to the foundations, and then build myself up again. It did not matter that an unpleasant treatment might have good results, because good results which

stemmed from a bad event would be cancelled out by this event. I
could not accept the illogical idea of a good thing emanating from a
bad, for instance a cornerstone resting safely on rubble despite the
evident fact that this could happen.

It is hardly necessary to point out the richness of architectural, spatial
and geometrical images in this reasoning.

The patient wanted to put a bolt on his door. In case it would not fit
the bolt-hole he replaced the latter with a bigger one. But he then
noticed it was now higher than before, although of the same diameter.
'I said to myself', he reported, 'that logically, because it is higher, it
ought to be wider and so I enlarged the hole'. There were more
difficulties and more mathematical considerations, and eventually he
ended up with a massive hole in the door and in the wall.

> 'Planning is everything for me in life', he went on, 'I wouldn't upset
> my plan for anything. I would rather upset my life. It is a taste for
> symmetry, for regularity that attracts me in planning. Life has no
> regularity or symmetry, and for that reason I manufacture my own
> reality. I attribute all my energies to my brain.
>
> What I am going to say may seem fantastic, but there it is. My state
> of mind consists of having no faith in anything except theory. I don't
> believe in the existence of anything until I have demonstrated it. For
> example, a woman's body has an effect on a man. Why? This is
> something that I doubt because I cannot prove it. I don't see myself
> giving way to such things, being carried away and relying only on my
> impressions. I would feel as if I were in the air, and that would be
> illogical.'

In the street, however, he was sometimes struck with the appearance
of a woman. He would then return to his house, sit down on a chair,
cross his arms and take up a position as symmetrical as possible to
reflect on the event. He would try to solve the problem of why a
woman's body made a particular impression on a man. He hoped that
it could all be explained 'by mathematics, medicine and sexual impressions'. It was in this manner that he sought an answer. He wondered
whether the human body cannot be reduced to geometry and therefore
whether the highest form of beauty did not consist in having a
spherical body, this being the perfect form.

He wrote:

> I want to examine my sexual impressions, even though this is a
> formidable problem, because the more I try to analyse these in terms
> of similar impressions, sub-impressions for instance, I only end up by
> deriving more impressions. And so it goes on.

He thought about what it would be like if he left hospital. He would become perplexed; his spatial thought, uniquely adapted to things which were durable and immobile, was totally incapable of taking in the slightest change. Here is his train of thought: 'I imagine myself leaving here. It is essential that I still keep some impression of being here and for that to happen I have to have something which represents my stay here'. And so when he left the hospital he took away with him all the bottles and all the empty boxes of pills used during his stay, and arranged them carefully in his house in order to have proof that he had been in the hospital and to have the impression that he was still there.

'I am always looking for immobility', he announced to us. 'I tend towards rest and immobilisation. I also have within me a tendency to prefer immobility in the things around me in my life. I like immovable objects, boxes and bolts, things that are always there, which never change. Stone is motionless, whereas the ground can move and inspires no confidence in me. I attach importance only to solidity. A train goes past on the embankment; the train doesn't exist for me: I want only to build the embankment.

The past is a precipice. The future is a mountain. It occurred to me that it would be a good idea to have a buffer-day between the past and the future. On this day I would do nothing at all. In this way I once went 24 hours without urinating.

I would like to recall my impressions of 15 years ago, to do away with time, to die with the same impressions that I was born with, to make circular movements, to stay in the same place, and not to be uprooted. All these things I would like.'

It would be hard to find a better example of the processes involved in purely spatial thought, which when liberated from the influence of the intuition which is indispensable to life tries to govern its own activity. We have seen the objectives which it sets out to achieve and the monstrous constructions at which it arrives. Can one imagine a better confirmation of those ideas of Bergson which were the point of departure of our analysis?

It should be added that when invited to write an account of all this our patient did so over numerous pages. Characteristically, he only mentioned objects, walls, boxes, bolts and bolt-holes; not one living person entered his description. One would say that his whole life was made up of solid and immovable objects.

It was equally clear that he never sought to combat his abnormal attitude. Not only did he accept it, but he continually tried to demonstrate its solid foundation with supra-logical and supra-rational arguments. He consulted us, not to be rid of his 'obsessions', but solely to 'rest', as he put it, in order to return to his bolts and other objects which were the mainstay of his life.

Madame Minkowska who examined this patient at length summarised her findings in the following way:

> *Life* in his case is opposed to planning;
> *instinct* to the brain;
> *feeling* to thought;
> the *faculty of penetration which synthesises* is opposed
> to analysis of infinite details;
> whereas we rely on *impressions*, he demands proof;
> *movement* is set against immobility;
> *events and people* are opposed to objects;
> *realisation* counters representation;
> *time* is in opposition to space;
> *succession* is contrasted with extension; and the *end*
> is set against the means.

In this scheme the first element in each contrasted pair (in italics) is deficient, the second element hypertrophied.

I subscribe to this analysis. One can interpret them as an atrophy of those factors which have to do with instinct, 'modelled on life', and a compensatory hypertrophy of everything which concerns intelligence, or as Bergson put it 'has as its principal object things which are inorganic solids, dead, or not renewed at any moment in time and which are characterised by a lack of natural understanding of life'.

Here is an account by another schizophrenic:

> Apart from my reason, which is intact, everything else is in complete disarray. I have suppressed my emotions as I have all aspects of reality. My body has an existence but there is no internal sensation in my life. I don't feel things any more. I don't have normal sensations. I make up for this lack of sensations with reason. Since my illness began I have suppressed the impression of time. Time doesn't matter any more. I can set aside an infinite amount of time to accomplish the most trivial act in my current life. I feel that I can reason quite well, but only in the absolute, because I have lost contact with life.

Another schizophrenic, in an advanced stage of her illness, passed the time making hats for herself. She had made 16 of them. One day, she lost two of them. As a form of retaliation against this she decided to break two of her mother's 16 cups.

Another patient, on being asked, after a visit to her mother, if she had been pleased to see her, replied: 'There was a lot of movement. I don't like that'.

One schizophrenic that I saw showed none of these obsessional phenomena, but needed to give some durable form to events in her life. She had collected newspapers and various scraps of paper relating to herself: 'This happened at this time and on this day (whereupon she indicated the exact hour and date) and I wrote this with a glass beside me which was exactly two centimetres from the paper I am writing on'. As she had done with the glass, on another occasion she took as her support, her witness as it were, any inanimate and immobile object which she found in front of her, e.g. a lamp.

One patient got hold of the idea that someone had put inside his stomach all the left-overs and all the scraps of a meal. He then interpreted everything that he saw in front of him in the light of this idea. His thoughts immediately took flight in the presence of an object, and he went into all the ramifications of how such an object could be related to him. The packet in which he received his copy of the newspaper *Figaro* made him think of the wrappings of all the other newspapers which had been delivered that day and then of all the wrappings of all the daily newspapers in France. One of his family had bronchitis and was bringing up phlegm. This led him to consider all the phlegm produced by patients in all the tuberculosis hospitals in France and then all the refuse of all these hospitals. He thought that all this had been put into his stomach. His son was shaving in front of him; the soldiers in the neighbouring barracks must therefore be shaving and then he thought about how the whole regiment must be doing it. A ticket for the Metro made him think of all railway tickets, Metro tickets, bus tickets and tram tickets that had ever been issued. The individual appearance of an object, event or person was thus wiped out. His thoughts took flight into infinite space with no boundaries.

One young patient with such morbid rationalisations spent a lot of time and energy setting up a programme for allocating his time minute by minute. He would set aside two minutes for washing himself before each meal. The whole plan was a failure as he could not carry it out. The same patient tried to keep his bottles of pills, so as to have a trace of things which would otherwise vanish with time. One day he was annoyed with himself because he felt well, when according to his calculations he should have felt tired. 'It's not logical', he told us.

All these observations have also been made by other writers on the subject. But I hope that I have been able to view them from a new angle, to group them in a more adequate way and therefore to promote a better understanding of them . . .

We cannot imitate the states of mind described by our patients, and so, when we try to deepen our theoretical and practical understanding of the human personality, we need not be afraid of applying our own instincts and our own intuition to the task.

Jacques Lacan (1900–81)

Jacques Lacan is regarded as the father of French psychoanalytical thinking. He trained in mainstream psychiatry and his doctorate thesis was supervised by Gaétan de Clérambault. After the Second World War he became a cult figure in French intellectual circles, mixing Freudian ideas with social comment. As with many French intellectuals, he founded an ephemeral one-man movement with many followers, who have dwindled sharply since his death.

The following extract from his thesis contains one of the clearest expositions of a psychogenic psychosis, the life history of the patient whom he calls Aimée, after the heroine of her own romantic autobiography, which is described affectionately and with insight.

The 'case of Aimée' stands as a sensitive and understandable rendering of the links between a certain personality and a certain psychotic development.

The case of Aimée, or self-punitive paranoia

J. Lacan (1932)

(Second Part, Le cas Aimée ou la paranoia d'auto-punition, of *De la Psychose Paranoiaque dans ses Rapports avec la Personalité*. Le François: Paris)

This paper examines the theoretical basis and the developmental origins of paranoid psychosis in terms of the personality development of a single case presented in detail . . .

Case history

The assassination attempt. On 10 April at eight o'clock in the evening Mme Z., a celebrated Parisian actress, arrived at the theatre where she was playing that evening. She was accosted at the stage-door by a stranger, who asked her: 'Are you Mme Z?' When she replied in the affirmative, the stranger, according to Mme Z., assumed a different facial expression, quickly took a knife out of her handbag and, with a look of hatred, raised her arm ready to strike her. Mme Z. tried to protect herself by seizing the blade, in the course of which she severed two tendons in her hand. By this time, the stranger had been overcome by two stagehands and the police were called. The stranger, whom we shall call Aimée from now on, was taken to the prison of Saint-Lazare, where she was kept for two months before being transferred to the Asylum of Saint-Anne.

On initial questioning Aimée explained her behaviour by saying that the actress had been instigating 'scandal' against her. According to Aimée, she had been mocking and menacing her for a number of years. Her accomplice in these acts of persecution was a famour writer, P.B., who had disclosed various incidents of her personal life in his novels.

Patient's life situation. Aimée was aged 38 at the time of this incident. She had been born in the Dordogne of a peasant family. She had two sisters and three brothers, one of whom had risen to become a teacher. She was currently employed as an administrator in one of the railway companies, and had been in this job since the age of 18. She was married to an employee of the same company, but for the last six years they had led separate lives, and she lived alone. She had one son, who lived with his father, but whom she saw regularly.

Previous forensic and psychiatric history. Six years before, she had been a voluntary patient in another psychiatric hospital. She had remained there for six months and the following extracts from her case-notes give some idea of her condition at that time: 'Psychiatric disorder of one year's duration . . . People in the street make insulting remarks, accuse her of extraordinary vices; people around her say all sorts of evil things about her; the whole town of Melun knows about her behaviour and regards her as depraved . . . Evidence of mental disorder, delusions of persecution and jealousy, illusions, misinterpretations, grandiose ideas, hallucinations, excitement, incoherence . . .' She was released after six months at the request of her family, although 'not cured'.

About a year before the present incident she was reported to the police by a communist journalist for continually pestering him to release copies of articles in which, she claimed, he had drawn attention to her grievances against a certain famous writer. Five months previously she was again reported to the police, this time for assaulting an employee of a publishing house which had rejected a manuscript. On this occasion she was not arrested, but merely reprimanded by the police . . .

Mental state on admission. By the time she was transferred to hospital the conviction attached to her delusions had completely disappeared. She was well orientated, had no intellectual impairment, showed no evidence of thought disorder and her attention was unimpaired. When recalling the themes of her delusions she felt ashamed and realised that they were ridiculous . . . However, her emotional response during the initial interviews, particularly the detached manner in which she referred to the victims of her assaults, suggested a lack of sincerity and even of dissimulation in her responses . . . In subsequent interviews she became more trusting and at this point it became apparent that, although her delusions had lost their intellectual appeal, some of them still evoked emotion. For example, she might say: 'I did that because someone wanted to kill my child'. The grammatical form in which she recounted the reasons for her behaviour, her defiant manner – head held high, arms crossed, trembling and hushed voice – and particularly the pallor which came over her face at such times, all suggested that they still exercised a powerful influence over her.

There were other signs which could not be taken for mere reticence: regular gaps in her memory, for example, and misunderstandings, consistent with the continued influence of delusional themes.

Development and content of delusions. Aimée's delusional state illustrated almost the entire range of paranoid themes. There were delusions of persecution, expressed through ideas of jealousy and prejudice. There were delusions of grandeur, with dreams of escaping to a better life and notions of having a grand mission to accomplish. Eventually she showed systematised erotomania attached to a royal personage. There were no hypochondriacal delusions, however, and no beliefs about being poisoned.

It was possible to date the onset of her psychiatric condition to when she was aged 28, ten years prior to her current admission. At that time she had been married for four years, was still working in the same office as her husband and had just become pregnant.

The first manifestation was a vague feeling, on her part, that colleagues at work were against her. They seemed to be criticising her work unduly, maligning her behaviour and saying unkind things to her. Later, passers-by in the street seemed to be whispering about her and showing their contempt for her. She noticed allusions to herself in newspapers. She was puzzled at the time by these incidents: 'Why do people behave like this? They must want my child inside me to die. If my child does not survive they will be to blame'.

The depressive element in all this is clear. She later wrote: 'During my pregnancies I felt sad. My husband would reproach me with this; this would cause a row; and then he would accuse me of having been with another man before I knew him. This caused me a lot of pain . . .'

She reacted in an aggressive manner. One day she slashed the tyres of a colleague's bicycle. One night she threw a jug of water at her husband's head; another time she threw an iron at him.

Her child was born dead. It was a girl, asphyxiated by having the cord around its neck. She was devastated. She blamed it all on her enemies, and in particular on a woman who for three years had been her best friend. This woman, who worked in a distant town, telephoned soon after her delivery to find out how she was. Aimée thought this strange, and her hostility crystallised from that moment.

A second pregnancy brought a return of her depressive state. She gave birth to a healthy child this time, a son, and devoted herself to looking after him. She breast-fed him until he was 14 months old, and during this period she became hostile and querulous, making all sorts of misinterpretations. She provoked a scene with the driver of a car which she considered had passed too close to the child's pram.

Her husband discovered that she was secretly planning a trip to America. When he confronted her with this information she said she was going to make her fortune there as a novelist. She said she would abandon her child, but then changed her mind, and said the trip was for his benefit.

This was the time of her first stay in a psychiatric hospital, after which she was better but 'not cured' according to the hospital records.

Following her discharge she refused to go back to work or even stay in the same town because, as she said, the persecution had made it unbearable. She obtained a transfer of her job to Paris and from that time onwards she became progressively preoccupied with Mme Z., the actress whom she eventually stabbed. She became convinced that Mme Z. was endangering her son's life. She later recalled: 'One day at the office, while I was as usual wondering where the threats to my son's life came from, I heard someone mention Mme Z. and I knew then that she was the one who wished us harm'.

One cannot help noticing the flimsiness of her evidence against Mme Z. We enquired carefully among her colleagues for any mention by her of this actress, and all we were able to discover were vague remarks directed at 'theatre people in general . . .' Aimée had only seen the actress twice before the assassination attempt, once on the stage and once on the screen. She could not even remember, however, the name of the play or film, or even if it was a classical or modern piece. This was so extraordinary that we have to regard it as a selective amnesia, hiding her true emotions.

Over the next five years her misinterpretations increased in number.

These were not confined to the actress, but included photographs of the house where she was born and newspaper references to her son being killed. Other persecutors emerged over this period, including the actress, Sarah Bernhardt, and the writer whom she had asked a journalist to vilify. Another writer, P.B., assumed a prominent role. He was, according to her, the cause of her divorce, as she had come to love him. As with Mme Z., the entry of P.B. into her delusions was uncertain in time and vague in its logical development . . . She recalled subsequently: 'I couldn't believe that Mme Z. was working alone and so I came to the conclusion that someone important must be working alongside her'. She thought she had found allusions to herself in P.B.'s novels, and for this reason she identified the author as an accomplice of Mme Z. Later still she came to believe that a career in literature had been marked out for her, and then that she was an expert in chemistry. At other times she thought she must be someone important in Government circles, an influence on the morals of others 'like Krishnamurti'.

She went through a phase of soliciting men in the street and, although she would take them back to a hotel, her main motive was not sexual satisfaction but to satisfy 'a great curiosity concerning men's way of thinking . . .'

She then developed an erotomania centred on the Prince of Wales. She sent him poems, and avidly collected newspaper cuttings of trips abroad, but never tried to meet him. Her erotomania was entirely platonic in nature . . .

Several months before the assault and her arrest she became increasingly agitated and desperate. She felt she had to see her main enemy face to face. One month before the incident she bought a knife and by her own account, on the evening of her actual encounter with the actress, she was in a state of extreme arousal and frenzy.

Literary productions. Her main literary productions were two novels, both written in the eight months before her arrest. From a literary point of view the first is better than the second, but both are well written. [The heroine of the first novel is called Aimée. In the first chapter, entitled 'Spring', she is pictured in an idyllic setting, as a country girl in the age of chivalry, dreaming of marriage. In the second chapter, 'Summer', two strangers make their appearance. One is a 'courtesan' who destroys the innocent atmosphere and of whom Aimée feels intensely jealous. In the third chapter, 'Autumn', disaster strikes, as Aimée and her fiancé become the subject of gossip and scandal in the town. She responds by thinking purer and purer thoughts. In the last chapter, 'Winter', she dies, just after the strangers go away – [Synopsis, Tr.]

In the second novel, one of the most significant passages is this invective against 'women of the theatre':

> High class prostitutes are the scum of society. They undermine it and destroy it. They make other women the slaves of society and ruin their reputation.
>
> Coming out of the theatre one night I saw a procession go by. The main figure in this was an old hag whose thighs must have been entered by millions over the years. There she was with her retinue of parasites, procurers and pimps, in the form of journalists. Her flabby body was perched on top of one of the carriages. Beauty, I heard one of her followers say to another, lies in the coccyx; generosity in the groin; intelligence in the little toe.
>
> I was told that this was how things went on round here. All I could see was a she-wolf made up to be a queen; following her there was an evil goddess wearing a dog-skin; then came the rest of the retinue poisoning the air with their foul breath; bringing up the rear was a she-goat who had just come out of the National Theatre with a wet rose in its mouth, all sticky and with a wig on its horns, whom the journalists were making eat all the pretty flowers in Paris.
>
> Poets came up one by one to talk to the old hag. Passers-by would grab hold of her thighs and the owner of the main newspaper in the city had his way with her in front of everyone. I couldn't go on. The procession stopped me. I asked people what the whole thing meant, but no one would tell me. It must be a secret of the theatre, something to do with the formalities of society: the motto was Honour and Nationhood.
>
> It really is too crude, Madame, but you do it nonetheless. You would never regard it as sinful. The whole thing is like a flying brothel, the sort of thing you can buy in special bookshops.

Diagnosis. The most striking aspect of the whole case is the delusional state. It was systematised, and its two main features were the accompanying emotion (predominantly anxiety), and the peculiar way in which it developed, particularly with regard to the seemingly casual choice of victim.

We can first of all exclude organic dementia, acute confusional state and dementia paranoides, as there was no evidence of intellectual impairment. Similarly, we can rule out both a chronic hallucinatory delusional state . . . and paranoid schizophrenia, because there were no hallucinations to suggest the former and no disturbance of ideation or affectivity to support the latter . . . Could it be a manic-depressive psychosis? Although Aimée was depressed during her first admission to hospital, her mood was not strikingly abnormal during the current admission and we cannot therefore attribute her entire condition to a manic-depressive psychosis . . .

We are therefore compelled to place Aimée's psychosis among the large body of conditions labelled paranoid psychoses. She fits the usual criteria perfectly: egocentricity, logical development from false premises and gradual use of defence mechanisms to consolidate it . . . Of the various types of paranoid psychoses one of the most well defined is that described by Sérieux and Capgras – a misinterpretative delusional state. Aimée fits this description very well. The only unusual features were the lack of any feeling of injustice and the absence of a sense of exaltation, both of which are common in misinterpretative delusional states, and the presence of a feeling of self blame which is uncommon in these states. Aimée believed that her child was being harassed because she herself deserved to be punished. Another unusual feature was the fact that the persecution was not entirely 'centrepetal', in that the child was the focus of some of the imagined threats . . .

In the next section we shall examine the actual way in which the psychosis developed.

Discussion

Does Aimée's psychosis represent an organic process? In order to elucidate the psychotic mechanisms, we shall first of all examine those phenomena which are primitive or elementary . . . These comprise symptoms which express the determining factors of the psychosis . . . In our case the role of the puerperium was clinically obvious. The two initial thrusts of the delusional state both occurred during her two pregnancies. In addition, one should consider her thyroid dysfunction which may have contributed to the initial psychiatric disorder, and one should also note that she abused the thyroid medication. In the established phase of her delusional state her menstrual rhythm determined the fluctuations in her anxiety level . . . Let us now examine the primitive mental symptoms which seem to have been caused by these organic factors . . . We can group them into four types:

(1) *Oneiroid states*, often coloured by anxiety; (2) *incomplete perceptions*; (3) *misinterpretations*; and (4) *illusions of memory* . . . Oneiroid states are those states of altered consciousness which resemble dreams. In our patient dreams played a major role in her mental life even before her first admission. Quite often, after the delusional state had set in, her

morbid mental state would begin as a dream and persist for several hours into her waking life. For example, on one occasion, she feared the arrival all morning of a telegram announcing her son's death; she had dreamed this the previous night and the belief had carried over into her waking state . . . Associated with these are atypical modifications, more or less in larval form, of perceptual structure . . . Misinterpretations are characterised by their selectivity, the sense of compulsion with which they arrest our attention, and the personal significance which they convey . . . Illusions of memory result from a weakening of the power of remembering which produces an invented image – whether itself the product of a perceptual association, a dream or a delusional complex – in place of a true memory image . . .

Our concept of the psychopathology of misinterpretative delusional states differs from the classical account by putting more weight on a 'psychasthenic' origin, that is to say that the social components of perception and memory are selectively affected. The classical account puts most weight on a disorder of reasoning . . . Our account has the advantage that one can link these misinterpretative states with certain organic states . . . But can one explain Aimée's delusional state in the light of the organic factors which were identified – the puerperium, thyroid dysfunction, abuse of thyroid medication, the menstrual cycle? Organic psychiatrists tend to regard a delusional system as the intellectual elaboration of organically-determined phenomena. Its structure, according to them, is of little importance. We cannot accept this formulation. We believe that the primitive phenomena discussed above (oneiroid state, incomplete perceptions, misinterpretations, illusions of memory) cannot explain how a delusional system can become established or account for its particular organisation. In our view the crucial factor lies in the personality of the subject, and this allows us to regard the development of the psychosis as a process disorder.

Does Aimée's psychosis represent a reaction to a vital conflict and emotionally-determined traumas? In order to answer this question we carried out a detailed enquiry of her background and personality from numerous sources. The most prominent traits and incidents were as follows:

As a young child, she was, by all accounts, very strong-willed. She was the only one in the household who could stand up to a tyrannical father. She was regarded by her parents as the brightest child and the only one most likely to succeed in life. She derived various privileges from this status. For example, her underwear was of better quality than that of her sisters, a fact which her sisters bitterly resented, and still did when interviewed years later . . .

The person who was responsible for her favourable treatment within the family was her mother. This led to an intense emotional bond between the two of them. Aimée said later 'We were like two friends' and often regretted ever having left her side. Her mother, moreover, had always been a suspicious person. On one occasion, for example, a neighbour had predicted that one of her cows which was ill would not get better. When the beast died, her mother accused her neighbour of having wished its death and of having poisoned it . . .

One trait, in particular, was noticeable from an early age. She was always slow and late for things. She was never ready at the same time as the others. This, as Janet pointed out, is typical of those who develop psychasthenic symptoms . . .

She was always rich in imagination, as could be seen in her adolescent writings. These were notable for a certain quasi-erotic precocity, with themes of her being a child of nature and accounts of passionate experiences . . .

At the age of 17 there were the first signs of a deficiency in psychological functioning. Until this time she had been top of the class at school and she thus obtained entry to a Teachers Training College. But within a short while of being there she received a minor setback and gave up the course. We can consider this too as evidence of a *professional abulia* or lack of will, within Janet's concept of psychasthenia. This is often associated with another symptom, which was to be quite marked throughout her adult life, that of a *need for moral direction*. One of her teachers commented at this period: 'Just when you think you know her, she escapes you'. He considered her a born liar.

After her return from Teachers Training College she decided on a career in administration. At this time, also, a close girl-friend died of pneumonia, and this affected her deeply.

We should not leave the period of infancy and adolescence without mentioning an incident which achieved almost a 'quasi-mythical value' in the family. The family were out for a walk in the country, and at some point Aimée was left behind because she was arranging her hair. In an attempt to catch up she took a short cut across a field and was chased by a bull. The incident recurred often in her dreams and in her writings . . .

Aimée's first contact with the wider world was in a provincial town far away from her birthplace. She lived there with her older sister who had married an old man when she was only 15. Aimée was soon dominated by this sister, whose influence on her was even more striking later in her life. The most significant event at this stage, however, was her first love affair. Her seducer appears a comic figure in retrospect. He was a small-town Don Juan and a poet in a group of 'regional artists'. At first Aimée found his advances repulsive, but she later gave in, and was then told that it was all a game to him. She left soon afterwards to work in another town, but he remained in her thoughts for three years. She wrote numerous letters to him and gave up all social life to devote her thoughts to him. At the end of these three years her emotions suddenly turned to hate. She later referred to him in this way: 'He can drop dead, for all I care. Don't talk to me about this chap, this ill-mannered lout . . .'

The next phase of her life, which lasted for four years until her marriage, was marked by a close friendship with a female colleague at work. This girl came of a noble family, but her branch of it had fallen on hard times. Despite this the girl behaved as if she were intellectually and morally superior to those around her. Aimée was first of all overwhelmed by this friend with her social airs and domineering attitude. Later, however, she began to keep, as she put it, 'a secret garden' within herself. Later still, she became irritated with her and the other girls in the circle: 'Women are only interested in gossip, intrigue and their own narrow lives', she wrote. She noticed at this time that her attitude and way of thinking were closer to a man's and recalled: 'I had an intense curiosity about men's minds . . .'

Aimée then married one of her colleagues, who offered her the chance of moral stability and practical security. The husband was a ponderous man, totally opposed to anything vain, decorative or creative. Her behaviour, in this respect, annoyed him intensely, and together with her sexual frigidity this led to marital rows. Both parties were jealous of the other. Aimée's reaction was predictable. She became retarded, 'abulic' and contrary in her behaviour. If asked to go for a walk, she would make any excuse to stay at home but, once out, she would prolong it for hours. Eight months after her wedding, however, something happened which was probably the most decisive event in her life. Her elder sister, the one with whom she had lived after leaving home, became a widow, and took up residence with Aimée and her husband. From our discussions with this sister it is quite clear that she had an immense influence on Aimée. She would give advice on everything and before long was the dominant member of the household. Aimée, as a result, became more and more estranged from her husband. Because her character was both sensitive and psychasthenic she could neither give in completely to her sister nor take refuge in daydreams. She experienced the situation as a moral humiliation. Her personality was such that she could not react simply with a combative attitude, which would be the typical paranoid response. The sister's most powerful weapon against Aimée was not so much her authority as Aimée's own conscience, for Aimée could recognise her sister's value, her virtues and her concern. It was this combination of the struggle to resist the sister's authority, and the recognition of her sister's qualities and her own humiliation, which formed the roots of her psychosis. In the town, it was common knowledge that her sister had supplanted her. Far from denying this or fighting it, Aimée would glady admit the fact . . .

The actual mechanism by which her sister became transformed into her 'enemy' will be dealt with in the next section. Before concluding this section, however, we shall contrast the main features of a typical paranoid personality with those found in Aimée.

Paranoid personalities are essentially proud and vain, whereas Aimée was both self-conscious and prone to crises of moral uncertainty. The former are distrustful in all situations, whereas our patient was intermittently anxious. The overriding psychological deficit in paranoid personalities is that of false judgement. In Aimée's case the problem is better regarded as one of an abundance of imagination which affects faculties such as judgement but which maintains some link with reality. Her faulty reasoning is a secondary effect, resulting from a primary emotional disorder, and in particular her *morbid conscience*.

Aimée's psychosis is based on self-punitive mechanisms which dominate her personality structure. Before embarking on the complex issues involved in this argument we should consider what is meant by personality functions. They consist of two sorts of reactions to events. There are those which have a social component and which play a part in the general well-being of those around them. Others are more concerned with maintaining the well-being of the subject in the face of judgements from others. There is a conscious aspect to each of these sets of functions and this means that they are intentional. The new discipline of psychoanalysis has thrown much light on the unconscious aspects of personality and on the distortions which appear to us as conscious intentional reactions.

It is not our primary aim here to consider whether the methods of

psychoanalysis, undoubtedly of value in many areas of psychopathology, can be applied to psychosis. We do not believe that one can apply
psychoanalytical methods to psychosis just because they have been
useful elsewhere. In our view it is justifiable to use psychoanalytical
principles, but in the rest of the discussion we hope to show that
Aimée's psychosis can be regarded as *psychogenic* purely by observing
the psychosis itself . . .

The first point to note, in support of a psychogenic cause of Aimée's
psychosis, is the fact that her symptoms disappeared abruptly on the
20th day of her imprisonment. She was 'cured', and remained cured for
the year and a half that we observed her in hospital. Perhaps we should
take heed of the old maxim, that *the nature of the cure will show you the
nature of the illness*. The way in which her symptoms remitted was
unlike that seen in organic, schizophrenic, depressive or manic conditions. These resolve slowly, with frequent oscillations, and then only
partially. In Aimée's case the entire delusional system evaporated
rapidly. Usually, cures of this sort are only seen in one set of circumstances – in subjects with delusional states based on passion who
have accomplished the murder of the person who is the object of the
delusion. Such subjects experience a characteristic relief accompanied
by an immediate resolution of all their delusional convictions. In
Aimée's case, however, the aggressive act against the actress did not
result in immediate relief; she obtained no satisfaction in contemplating
her victim's plight. Nor did her delusions disappear immediately; they
persisted for another 20 days. But it did seem to us as if something had
changed as a result of her attack. She was made to undergo a punishment: in prison she was forced into the company of criminals; she was
in daily contact with their behaviour, opinions and cynical remarks on
her situation; and she had to suffer the scorn and desertion of everyone
she knew. For this reason, there were similarities between Aimée's
case and delusional states of passion. Her delusional state did eventually resolve and she did later experience relief. The delay in her case
represented the time it took for her to become aware of her punishment
and it was at the point that 'relief' came . . .

We have thus tentative evidence for a *self-punitive* trait or a *feeling of
culpability* in Aimée's case which underlay the development of her
psychosis. This hypothesis explains other features of the case, for
instance the content of her delusions. Her persecutors were trying to
harm her child 'in order to punish the mother'. On one occasion, when
asked why she had believed her child was being threatened, she

replied: 'To punish me, because I did not accomplish what I set out to do . . .'

A second striking feature of the case is the peculiar nature of her persecutors. There were several of them, but none had any relationship in real life with Aimée. This fact highlights the purely symbolic significance of these persecutors. They were, we might say, second, third and successive moulds of a *prototype*. This prototype has two aspects, emotional and representational.

The emotional power of the prototype is to be found in the real life of our patient. We suggested earlier that it mainly derived from her feelings for her elder sister, on account of whom Aimée had suffered moral humiliation and reproaches to her conscience. To a lesser degree it also derived from envy of her close girlfriend, who represented for Aimée the social adaptation and superiority which she herself felt she lacked.

The representational value of her persecutors is obvious. The sense of freedom and social ease which writers, actresses and women of the world reputedly possess were the very qualities which she herself dreamt of obtaining. They were her ideal, and at the same time the object of her hate. In striking the actress, Aimée struck her externalised ideal, in the same way as someone driven by passion strikes the unique object of their hate and their love. In Aimée's case, however, the value of the object was purely symbolic, and the act did not by itself lead to relief. But by the same blow which made her guilty in the eyes of the law, she received a blow to herself. When she had time to comprehend this, she experienced the satisfaction of a desire accomplished; her delusions, rendered ineffective by this realisation, vanished.

In this way we have, it would seem, demonstrated that the nature of the cure reveals the nature of the illness.

What of the link between the personality of the patient and the fundamental mechanisms by which her delusions arose? Aimée is best described as possessing traits of two clinical personality disorders: the psychasthenic and the sensitive. Obsessional scruples, continual doubts about ethical matters and internal moral conflicts are among their prominent features. Unlike someone with a normal personality, where mild organic insults and life events leave a relatively small trace, soon compensated for, someone with a self-punitive personality reacts entirely differently. The emotional and intellectual consequences of such events are not easily accommodated; they become fixed and persist. Thus, the development of a psychosis, such as we have described in the case of Aimée, is to be regarded as an effect of organic insults and life events acting on a pre-existing psychological anomaly. The psychological anomaly we regard as a disorder of personality, and our whole concept of psychotic development in this case can be termed *psychogenic*.

Index

Abraham, K., wish fulfilment 44
abstraction, disorder of 189
abulia, professional 221
activity
    level of physical, in simple
        schizophrenia 28
    mental, insufficiency of 51–8, 117
acute delusional states 169
    misinterpretations based on 179–80
acute insanity, differentiation from
        hebephrenia 156
acute stages of schizophrenia, prognosis
        of 64–5, 69
Adler, A., 126
affect
    in catatonic dementia praecox 39
    delusional ideas and 117
    dream content and 43–4
    flattening of, prognosis of 67, 70
    in mild dementia praecox 15
    in simple schizophrenia 28
    suspiciousness as an 129
    see also delusional mood states;
        depressed mood; emotions; manic
        mood
affective dementia in schizophrenia 200
affective psychosis, delusional states of
        passion secondary to 183–4
affective symptoms
    in acute schizophrenia 64
    at onset of dementia praecox 17, 18–19
    see also anxiety; depression;
        manic-depressive illness
age, development of delusions and 130–1
age of onset
    dementia praecox 22–3
    hebephrenia 154
    paranoid insanity 156
    simple schizophrenia 30–1

agnosias, paralogical thought disorder
        in relation to 77
Aimée, the case of (self-punitive
        paranoia) 213–26
    the assassination attempt 213–14
    development and content of delusions
        215–17
    diagnosis 218–19
    life situation 214
    literary productions 217–18
    mental state on admission 214–15
    previous forensic and psychiatric
        history 214
    psychotic development 219–26; organic
        influences 219–20; reactive
        components 220–3; self-punitive
        personality structure and 223–6
alcohol, effect on schizophrenics of 63
alcoholic dementia, differentiation from
        simple schizophrenia 32
alcoholic psychoses, delusional
        perception in 107
alogical thought disorder in
        schizophrenia, organic nature of 77–8
amentia
    anxiety associated with 39
    differentiation from catatonic dementia
        praecox 38
amnesias, word 75
amnesic syndrome, perplexity associated
        with 82
Anglade, D., dissociated patients 190
anthropology, influence on
        psychopathology of 137–8
'anti-psychiatry' movement 2, 6, 139–40
anxiety
    in amentia 39
    distinction of perplexity from 79
    misinterpretation and 106

anxiety *continued*
  perplexity associated with 80, 81
  in reactive disorders 82
  in schizophrenia 69
  in self-punitive paranoia 218, 219
anxious perplexity 80
apathy
  in catatonic dementia praecox 39
  in severe dementia praecox 17, 19
  in simple schizophrenia 28–9, 30
aphasia, relationship of schizophrenic
    speech and thought disorders to 5,
    75–6, 78, 138
'apparent psychosis' 128
apperceptive dementia, Weygandt's
    concept of 49, 189
'arrest of the flow of existence' 83–4, 86
Aschaffenburg, G., 61, 118, 120
Asperger's syndrome, relationship to
    schizophrenia of 2, 3
association, disturbance of 68, 86, 113,
    193
  prognosis of 64, 70
  see also dissociation of and between
    mental functions
association psychology 86, 130
asthenic personality, paranoid delusional
    formation in 137
ataxia, intrapsychic, *see* intrapsychic
    ataxia
athymhormia, juvenile 201
attention, disturbance of 29, 40, 189
  see also consciousness
autism
  Bleuler's concept of 191, 193
  existential analysis 85, 88
  Minkowski's concept of (loss of vital
    contact with reality) 8, 188–93
  in relation to schizophrenia 2–3
  see also reality; withdrawal from the
    external world
automatisms
  in mental deficiency 49
  secondary nature of 67
awareness
  delusional 105, 107
  in mild dementia praecox 14–15
  in simple schizophrenia 28
  see also consciousness; self-awareness

behaviourism 3, 7
Being and Time 138
belonging, disordered sense of 124–5
Bergson, Henri, 191, 193–4, 209, 210
Berze, Joseph, 3, 51–8, 116–17
  depersonalization 53
  disturbances of consciousness 52–3
  insufficiency of mental activity 51–2,
    117

personality change 54
split personality 55–8
thought fusion 114
Bilz, R., comparative behaviour 140
Binswanger, Ludwig, 4, 83, 138
  existential analysis of schizophrenic
    symptoms 5, 83–8
Binswanger, Otto, 83
biological sciences in relation to
    psychiatry 89, 140
Birnbaum, K., 120
Bleuler, Eugen, 25, 59–74, 85, 137, 190
  concept of autism 191, 193
  delusions 66, 70, 120, 124, 126, 130
  disturbances of consciousness 52–3, 55,
    66, 69, 70
  introduction of the term schizophrenia
    2, 4, 59
  personality deterioration 54
  prognosis of schizophrenia 59–74
  schizophrenic dementia 63–4, 67, 72–3,
    195, 200
  splitting of psychic functions 55, 59, 86
blind, persecutory delusions 126
bodily symptoms, *see* physical
    symptoms
body weight, changes in 21, 68
Bonhoeffer, K., exogenous reactions 118
brain damage, *see* organic brain damage
brain stem, thought disorders and 77, 78
Breuer, J. 42
Buehler, Karl 135–6
Bumke, O. 119, 120

Capgras, Joseph, misinterpretative
    delusional states, 7, 167, 168–81, 219
Capgras syndrome 168
catalepsy, secondary nature of 67
catatonia
  cerebral oedema in severe 68, 71
  Chaslin's (P.) concept of (discordant
    motor insanity) 147, 152–3, 157–8
  in manic-depressive illness 64–5
  prognosis of 60, 64, 69
  as a secondary phenomenon 67
  speech disorders in 76
  Stransky's (E.) diagnosis of a case of
    38–9
cerebral dysfunction, delusions caused by
    130
  see also organic brain damage; organic
    cerebral disorders
cerebral hemispheres, imbalance between
    3, 4, 8, 37
cerebral oedema in severe catatonia 68, 71
cerebral syphilis, differentiation from
    hebephrenia 156
  see also general paralysis of the insane

Chaslin, Philippe, 147
  discordant insanity 6, 147–58, 189–90
  mental confusion 192
  schizophrenic dementia 154, 155–6, 195
children
  development of paranoia 131
  normal speech development 49
  primitive modes of thinking 99, 131
cognitive therapy of delusional
  symptoms 7
comparative behaviour research,
  psychopathology and 140
complexes, role in development of
  dementia praecox 47
compulsive disorders of abnormal
  significance ('symbolic awareness')
  100–2, 103
confabulatory delusional states (délires
  d'imagination) 6–7, 159–67
  a case history 163–6
  medicolegal consequences 166–7
  origin of 159–62, 167
conflicts, inner, formation of delusions
  and 124–6
confusion 68–9
  assessment in 65
  mental, evolution of the term 192
  remission of 69
  see also consciousness, clouding of
connections, increased ability to form
  96–8
  see also reference/self-reference;
    significance, delusional perception of
Conrad, K.
  delusional perception 5, 99, 100
  Gestalt analysis 138
conscience, morbid, in self-punitive
  paranoia 223
consciousness
  clouding of 52–3; delusions secondary
    to 118, 127
  disturbances of 3; Berze's views on 3,
    51–8; Bleuler's concept of 52–3, 55;
    Gross's views on 3, 36, 40;
    misinterpretations based on 179;
    prognosis of 66, 69, 70; Wernicke's
    concept of 36, 40
  dream, wish fulfilment and 43
  in mild dementia praecox 14
  see also attention, disturbances of;
    awareness; confusion
constitution, development of delusions
  and 128–9
criminal behaviour in simple
  schizophrenia 29
The Crisis in Psychology 136
culpability, feeling of 224–5
cyclothymic personality 129

de Clérambault, Gaétan Gatian
  erotomania 7, 182, 184–7
  psychoses of passion 7, 182–7
deaf, persecutory delusions 126
déjà vu experiences 109–10
délire collectif 167
délire d'interpretation, *see*
  misinterpretative delusional states
délires d'imagination, *see* confabulatory
  delusional states
delirium
  febrile, paranoid states in 127
  perplexity associated with 81
delusion-like ideas (secondary
  delusions) 169
  differentiation from genuine delusions
    105, 120
  origins of 117–19
delusional atmosphere, *see* delusional
  mood states
delusional awareness 105, 107
delusional ideas
  definitions 120
  differentiation from delusional
    misinterpretation 170
  genuine 105, 120
  in manic-depressive illness 117
  in misinterpretative delusional states
    173–4, 180–1
  prognosis of 69, 70
  sudden, *see* sudden delusional ideas
  see also delusions; grandiose ideas;
    ideas; hypochondriacal ideas;
    persecution, ideas of
delusional interpretation 105
delusional misinterpretations, *see*
  misinterpretations, delusional
delusional mood states (delusional
  atmosphere) 105, 116
  content of delusional perception and
    107
  'end of the world experience' 106,
    109
  thought disorder secondary to 115
delusional perception 5
  Gruhle's (H.) concept of 106–7
  Jaspers' (K.) concept of 105
  Kurt Schneider's concept of 107, 108
  Matussek's (P.) concept of 5–6, 89–103,
    138–9; compulsive disorders of
    significance ('symbolic awareness')
    100–2, 103; elaboration of a new
    perceptual context 96–8, 103;
    'framed' perceptual qualities 95–6,
    103; loosening of the conceptual
    context 90–3, 94, 95, 103; 'primary'
    102, 103; rigidity of perception 93–4;
    symbolic context and identification

Matussek's concept *continued*
  on the basis of similar qualities 100,
  103
  see also perception, disturbances of
delusional states 7, 169
  acute, *see* acute delusional states
  of passion, *see* passion, delusional
  states of
  systematized, *see* paranoia
  see also confabulatory delusional states;
  hallucinatory delusional states;
  misinterpretative delusional states
delusions
  Bleuler's (E.) concept of 66, 120
  causal explanations 116–17, 128–32;
  cerebral dysfunction 127, 130; in
  confabulatory delusional states 160,
  161, 162–4; constitution 128–9; in
  hallucinatory delusional states 160,
  161–2; life epoch 130–1;
  manic-depressive illness 129–30; in
  misinterpretative delusional states
  160–1, 162, 175–80; perceptual
  disorders 116–17, 160; regression to
  an earlier stage of development
  131–2; sexuality 130
  in Chaslin's (P.) paranoid insanity
  149–50
  cognitive therapy for 7
  definitions 119–20
  in dementia praecox 17, 18, 19, 21
  descriptive studies 105–17; functional
  approach 112–15; ontological
  approach 115–16; phenomenological
  approach 105–12
  Schmidt's (G.) review of German
  literature 104–34
  secondary change of primary 118;
  see also delusion-like ideas
  in self-punitive paranoia 215–17
  understandable explanations 120–8;
  external conflict 126–8; inner conflicts
  and emotions 124–6; personality
  disorder 120–4, 137
dementia
  affective, in schizophrenia 200
  alcoholic, differentiation from simple
  schizophrenia 32
  apperceptive, Weygandt's concept of
  49, 189
  in Chaslin's hebephrenia 155–6
  meaning of 35
  organic, *see* organic dementia
  pragmatic 200
  primary 33–4
  schizophrenic 18, 19–20, 21, 154;
  assessment of 63, 72–3; distinction
  from intellectual dementia 8,

193–201; nature of 63–4, 200–1;
  progress of 73
  see also intelligence
dementia paranoides 150
  see also paranoia; paranoid insanity
dementia praecox
  definition by Dide and Guiraud 201
  Kraepelin's concept of 1, 2, 13–24, 153,
  154, 188–9; age of onset 22–3; causes
  21–2, 23; differential diagnosis 23–4;
  milder form 13–16;
  psychopathological mechanisms 189,
  190; severe form 16–21; treatment 24
  problems of using the term 59, 154
  simple, *see* simple schizophrenia
  see also catatonia; hebephrenia;
  paranoia; schizophrenia
dementia sejunctiva 35–6
dementia simplex, *see* simple
  schizophrenia
depersonalization
  Berze's concept of 3, 53
  in manic-depressive patients,
  perplexity and 81
  in schizophrenia 53, 197
  see also self-awareness
depressed mood
  delusional ideas in 117
  misinterpretations based on 179–80
  in schizophrenia 17, 64, 69
  in self-punitive paranoia 215, 216,
  218–19
depression
  differentiation from hebephrenia 156
  perplexity associated with 80–1, 82
  see also manic-depressive illness
'depth psychology' 126
descriptive psychopathology 136–7
  see also delusions, descriptive studies
Dide, M., definition of dementia praecox
  201
Diem, Otto, description of simple
  schizophrenia 2, 3, 25–34
discordance 153, 189–90
discordant insanity 6, 147–58
  dementia in 154, 195
  discordance and 153
  hebephrenia 147–9, 154–6
  motor insanity or catatonia 147, 152–3,
  157–8
  paranoid insanity 147, 149–50, 156–7
  verbal insanity 147, 150–2, 157
disorientation
  in amnesic syndrome 82
  in general paralysis of the insane 196–7
  in schizophrenia/dementia praecox 14,
  18, 196, 197

disposition, time-course of schizophrenia and 62
dissociation between and within mental functions 4, 47, 190
  Minkowski's views on 194–5, 210
  Stransky's views on 4, 36, 37, 40–1
  see also association, disturbance of; discordant insanity; intrapsychic ataxia; splitting of psychic functions
The Divided Self 5, 83
'double book keeping' 112
dream-like states, *see* oneiroid states
dreams
  experiences turned into delusions 19, 180, 219–20
  psychology of 43–5
Dupré, Ernest, confabulatory delusional states 6–7, 159–67
dynamic mental functions 198–200
dynamism, meaning of 198

eating habits, deterioration of 19
echo symptoms in mental deficiency 49
elderly, development of delusions in 130–1
Elements of Semiology and Clinical Mental Conditions 147
emotions
  delusions derived from 118, 124, 130, 182–4
  inability to show 189
  maintenance of delusions and 7
  see also affect; affective symptoms; delusional mood states
'end of the world experience' 85, 106, 108–9, 114
endogenous misinterpretations 178–80
environment, perceived, *see* perceptual context
environmental (external) factors
  causing psychoses 126–8, 137
  prognosis of schizophrenia and 62–3, 70–1
  see also psychogenic psychoses; reactive neuroses
epilepsy
  delusions of self-reference in 106
  differentiation from hebephrenia 156
  in discordant insanity 154
epileptic twilight states
  delusional perception in 107
  'end of the world experience' 109
eroticism, ideas of 173, 181
erotomania 7, 182, 215, 217
  prodromal 186, 187
  pure 184–6
  secondary 186–7

errors, differentiation from delusional misinterpretation 170–1
'establishment of a relationship without cause' 106, 107, 109
Ewald, G. 126, 129
excitement, states of 18, 19, 20, 28
executive thinking 78
existential analysis
  of delusions 115–16
  by Ludwig Binswanger 5, 83–8, 138
existentialism 138
exogenous misinterpretations 175–8
'exogenous reactions' of Bonhoeffer, secondary delusions in 118
external factors, *see* environmental factors
extravagance and schizophrenia 83, 84, 86

fabricate, tendency to 162
  see also mythomania
factor X, Jung's (C.) 47, 48
fainting fits in dementia praecox 20
family
  background of schizophrenics 139
  distress caused by simple schizophrenia 31
Fankhauser, E. 129–30
flight of ideas, organic cause of 77
Foersterling, W. 127
folie communiquée 128
folie à deux 128, 167
folie imposée 128
folie transformée 128
folies raisonnantes 171
  see also reasoning, disorders of
'framed' perceptual qualities 95–6, 103
Freud, Sigmund 126, 137
  notion of wish reversal 125
  Weygandt's criticism of 4, 42–50
frontal lobe defects, speech and thought disorders in 76
Functional Analysis of Schizophrenia 114

Ganser's syndrome 38, 66
Gaupp, R., role of personality in delusional formation 120–2, 137
general paralysis of the insane
  delusional ideas in 117
  differential diagnosis 32, 156
  intellectual impairment of 195–201
General Psychopathology 136
geometry, morbid preoccupation with 206–10
Gestalt psychology applied to delusional perception 5–6, 89–103, 138–9
grandiose ideas
  in the elderly 131
  in general paralysis of the insane 117

grandiose ideas *continued*
  in misinterpretative delusional states
    173, 174, 181
  in schizophrenia 18, 19, 199
  secondary to persecutory delusions
    121–2
  in self-punitive paranoia 215
Gross, Otto, 35–6, 41, 47
  disturbances of consciousness 3, 36, 40
Gruhle, H. W., 125, 136
  déjà vu experiences and memory
    distortions 109–10
  delusional perception 98, 105–7, 114
  delusions in psychopathic personalities
    118
  speech disorders 76
Guiraud, P., definition of dementia
    praecox 201

hallucinations 14, 17, 21, 66
  delusions secondary to 118, 160
  differentiation from delusional
    misinterpretation 170
  in misinterpretative delusional states
    170
  prognosis of 69
hallucinatory delusional states 160, 161–2
hallucinatory insanity 153
harmony with life, feeling of 202–3
headache in schizophrenia 68
hebephrenia
  attenuated, Chaslin's (P.) 147–8, 156
  Chaslin's concept of 147–9, 154–6, 190
  'discordant insanity' and 6
  Kraepelin's view of 22
  similarity to simple schizophrenia 32,
    34
heboidophrenia 33
Hecker, E., hebephrenia 22, 32
Hedenberg, S., delusional ideas 98, 111,
    118
Heidegger, M., 83, 138
Helmchen, H., 140
hemispheres, cerebral, imbalance
    between 3, 4, 8, 37
Herschmann, H., mentally subnormal
    soldiers 127
Hesse, H., paranoid states 127
Heveroch, A., delusions of reference 112
Hippius, H., 140
Hoche, A., 45, 117, 119
Homburger, A., delusional formation in
    children 131
Hoppe, A., 119
Hughlings Jackson, J., 140
hypochondriacal ideas 17, 131
  in misinterpretative delusional states
    173, 181

hypochondriacal states, perplexity and 82
hysteria
  differential diagnosis 32, 38, 156
  perplexity in 82
  psychoanalytical theories of 42–3, 45,
    47
ideas
  of bodily influence 19
  delusional, *see* delusional ideas
  'interruption in the flow of' 29
  overvalued 120
  slowing down of 157–8
  use of the term 108
  see also eroticism, ideas of; grandiose
    ideas; hypochondriacal ideas;
    persecution, ideas of
ideational agnosias 77
identification on the basis of similar
    qualities 99–100, 103
  see also misidentifications
'ideo-affective association' 182, 183
illusions
  differentiation from delusional
    misinterpretation 170
  of memory 164, 219, 220
imagination
  creative, in confabulatory delusional
    states 160, 161, 162, 164
  erotomania based on 186, 187
  in self-punitive paranoia 221, 223
imaginings, delusional ideas as 107
influence, ideas of bodily 19
inner unity, loss of 17–18, 189, 190
instinct in relation to intelligence,
    Minkowski's (E.) views on 194–5, 210
institutions
  effects on behaviour of admission to 28,
    30
  types of cases admitted to 71–2
insufficiency of mental activity 51–8, 117
intelligence
  in hebephrenia 155
  in relation to instinct, Minkowski's (E.)
    views on 194–5, 210
  in schizophrenia 189, 195
  see also dementia
interpretation
  delusional 105
  false, differentiation from delusional
    misinterpretation 170–1
  see also misinterpretations
The Interpretation of Dreams 43
intrapsychic ataxia, Stransky's (E.) 4, 37,
    39–41, 154, 189–90
intrapsychic dysharmony, Urstein's (X.)
    154, 190
irritability in dementia praecox 17, 20

irritable personality, paranoid delusional
formation in 137
Iwanow-Smolensky, A. G. 130

Jahrreiss, W., definition of delusions 120
Janet, P., concept of psychasthenia 192,
221
Janzarik, Werner, trends in psycho
pathology 6, 135–43
Jaspers, Karl
delusions 104, 105, 112, 114, 120, 126
understanding psychology and 90, 136,
137
jealousy, ideas of 173, 181
Jossmann, P., 120
judgement
delusional 108
in dementia 195
Jung, C., 35, 38, 126
theories of dementia praecox 46–8
justice neurosis 128
juvenile athymhormia 201

Kahlbaum, K. L., 33, 153
Kahn, E., 125
Kant, Otto, views on delusional reality
98, 125–6
Kehrer, F., 123–4
Kisker, K., role of psychiatrists 142
Kleist, Karl, organic explanations of
schizophrenia 4, 5, 75–8, 130–1
Knigge, F., 127
Kolle, K., 110, 127–8, 129
Kraepelin, Emil, 2, 13, 136
definition of delusions 119
description of dementia praecox, *see*
dementia praecox, Kraepelin's
concept of
on litiginous paranoia 127
use of the word 'dementia' 35
view of paranoia 121, 126, 128–9, 131
Kretschmer, E., sensitive delusions of
reference 122–3, 137
Kronfeld, A., 114–15, 126
Kunz, H., schizophrenic change of
existence 115–16, 126

Lacan, Jacques, a case of psychogenic
psychosis 8, 213–26
Laing, R. D., 5, 83, 139
Lange, J.
delusional ideas 119, 120
personality traints of paranoid subjects
121, 124, 129
Langelueddeke, A., sensitive paranoia
124
language
barrier, persecutory delusions and 126

incoherent 157
see also speech disorders of
schizophrenia
latent schizophrenia 61
laughter, affectless 15
letter writing in mild dementia praecox 16
Levy-Bruehl, M., 100
lie, tendency to 162
see also mythomania
life epoch, development of delusions and
130–1
life events, adverse 8
see also psychogenic psychoses; reactive
neuroses
litiginous paranoia 127–8
Logre, Jean, confabulatory delusional
states 6–7, 159–67

mania
differentiation from hebephrenia 156
remission of 69
manic mood
delusional ideas in 117
swings in schizophrenia 69
manic-depressive illness
catatonic symptoms in 64–5
delusions in 117, 129–30
differentiation from dementia praecox
23
'end of the world experiences' 109
perplexity associated with 80–1
manneristic behaviour and schizophrenia
83, 84, 87
Marxist influences on psychiatry 139
Masselon, R., disorder of attention 189
Matussek, Paul, 4, 89
Gestalt psychology applied to
schizophrenia 5–6, 89–103, 138–9
Maxwell Jones, therapeutic community
139
Mayer-Gross, W., 106, 126, 130, 136
memory
delusional ideas as 107
distortions, schizophrenic 14, 20, 52,
109–10
hallucination of 164
ilusions of 164, 219, 220
in intellectual dementia 195, 198
in schizophrenic dementia 195
see also misidentification
menopause, progress of schizophrenia
and 73
menstruation
delusional states and 219, 220
in dementia praecox 20
excited behaviour and 18, 21
mental activity, insufficiency of 51–8, 117

mental functions
    dissociation of, *see* dissociation of and
        between mental functions
    slowing down of 68
mental subnormality
    development of paranoid delusional
        states in 126–7, 128
    diagnosis from dementia praecox 24
mescaline intoxication, perception in 94,
    100
Metzger, W., primitive thinking 99
Minkowski, Eugene, 4, 7–8, 85, 188–212
    differences between intellectual
        dementia and schizophrenic
        dementia 193–201
    spatial thought in schizophrenia 201–12
    vital contact with reality 188–93
misidentifications 99–100, 103, 109
    of people 100, 109
misinterpretations
    delusional: definition and
        identification of 164, 170–1;
        in misinterpretative delusional
        states 160–1, 174–5; in self-punitive
        paranoia 216–17, 219, 220
    endogenous 178–80
    exogenous 175–8
misinterpretative delusional states
    (délires d'interpretation) 7, 162, 167
    169–81
    characteristics of 160–1, 171–3
    definition of 171
    delusional ideas 173–4, 180–1
    delusional misinterpretations 160–1,
        174–5
    endogenous misinterpretations 178–80
    exogenous misinterpretations 175–8
    self-punitive paranoia 219, 220
    symptoms 173
mood, *see* affect
Mosbacher, F. W., 131
motives, explicability in terms of 110, 117
    see also understanding psychology
motor insanity, discordant, (catatonia)
    147, 152–3, 157–8
movement disorders in schizophrenia 49
muscular excitability 20, 67–8
mutism, secondary nature of 67
mysticism, ideas of 173, 181
mythomania 159, 162, 165, 167

negativism, secondary nature of 67
neologisms in discordant verbal insanity
    157
neurasthenia 33, 156
Neustadt, R., 128
nihilistic delusions 131
noo-psyche, Stransky's 4, 39, 40

obsessional behaviour in schizophrenia
    207–8
obsessional neuroses
    compulsive disorders of significance in
        101–2, 103
    delusional states of passion secondary
        to 183
    differentiation from hebephrenia 156
oedema in schizophrenia 68
oneiroid states (dream-like states) 219
    assessment in 65
organic brain damage
    delusional states and 127, 130
    patterns of bahaviour resembling
        symptoms of 39
    speech and thought disorders of,
        in relation to schizophrenic 75–8
organic cerebral disorders
    alogical thought disorder in 75–8
    delusional perception in 107
    perplexity associated with 81–2
    simple schizophrenia differentiated
        from 32
organic dementia
    clouding of consciousness 53
    schizophrenic dementia compared to 8,
        193–201
    simple schizophrenia differentiated
        from 33
organic psychoses
    differential diagnosis 24, 156
    secondary delusions in 118
overvalued ideas 120

painful stimuli, reactions to 39, 40–1
paralogical thought disorder, organic
    nature of 76–7, 78
paranoia (systematized delusional states;
    dementia paranoides)
    as an affective disorder 129–30
    differential diagnosis 23–4, 32–3, 156
    inner conflicts and emotions leading
        to 124–6
    litigious 127–8
    personality types predisposing to
        development of 120–4, 126, 128–9,
        137, 223–6
    psychogenic or reactive 126–8, 213–26
    self-punitive (the case of Aimée) 213–26
    subdivision of 6–7, 169
    see also delusions; delusional states;
        persecutory delusions
paranoid insanity, Chaslin's, (P.), 147,
    149–50, 156–7
paranoid personality 223
    development of paranoid psychosis
        from 120–2
paraphasias 75, 77

passion, delusional states of 182–4
abortive or attenuated 183
associated 183
prodromal 182–3
pure or autonomous 182, 183–4
secondary 182–3
see also erotomania
passion, psychoses of 7, 182–7
perception
delusional, *see* delusional perception
disturbances of 5–6; delusions as a
product of 106–7, 116–17; in
hallucinatory delusional states 160; in
self-punitive paranoia 219, 220
rigidity of 93–4
perceptual context (perceived
environment)
elaboration of a new 96–8, 103
loosening of components from 90–3,
94, 95, 103
perceptual qualities (*Wesenseigenschaft*),
'framed' 95–6, 103
perplexity, Störring's, (G.), views of 5,
79–82
in chronic organic reactions 81–2
definition of 79
in delirium 81
in hypochondriacal states 82
in manic-depressive illness 80–1
in psychasthenic personality disorder
82
in reactive mental disorders 82
schizophrenic 79–80
persecution, ideas of 17, 19
in misinterpretative delusional states
173, 181
reactive or psychogenic 126–7
relationship to delusions of grandeur
121–2
in self-punitive paranoia 215
personality
change: during the delusional
experience 111–12; in schizophrenia
3, 54
cyclothymic 129
functions 223
predisposing to development of
paranoia 120–4, 126, 128–9, 137, 223–6
schizoid 2–3
splitting of 3, 55–8
perverseness and schizophrenia 83, 84, 87
pharmacotherapy, psychopathology and
141
phobic neuroses, delusional states of
passion secondary to 183–4
physical symptoms
in Chaslin's discordant motor insanity
(catatonia) 158

in dementia praecox 20
misinterpretations based on 178–9
as primary symptoms of schizophrenia
67–8
Ploog, J. W., comparative behaviour
research 140
poverty, delusions of 131
pragmatic deficit in schizophrenia 200
pragmatic dementia 200
pregnancy, delusional states associated
with 215, 216, 219, 220
prejudice, age and 131
primitive people, modes of thinking in
99–100, 131–2
prisoners, paranoid reactions in 127
professional abulia 221
prototype persecutors 225
psychasthenia/psychasthenic personality
disorder
development of self-punitive paranoia
and 221, 223, 225
perplexity and 82
reality function 192
psychoanalytical theories
dream interpretations 43–5
of hysteria 42–3, 45, 47
of psychotic development 137, 223–4
of schizophrenia, Weygandt's
criticisms of 4, 45–8, 50
psychodynamic approaches to delusions
126
psychogenic (reactive) psychoses
the case of Aimée (Lacan) 8, 213–26
paranoid 126–8
perplexity associated with 82
psychopathic personality disorder,
delusional ideas in 118–19
psychopathology 90
of delusions 89
Janzarik's article on trends in 135–43
psychoses passionelles, *see* passion,
psychoses of
pupillary excitability 67, 68

quarrelsome or querulous paranoiac
personality type, delusional
development in 122–3

rage, remission of 69, 70
rational thinking 78
rationalisation, morbid 201–6, 211
Ratlosigkeit 79
see also perplexity, Störring's views of
reactions to painful stimuli 39, 40–1
reactive neuroses, perplexity associated
with 82
reactive psychoses, *see* psychogenic
psychoses

reactivity, mental, reduction in 20, 51, 52
reality
    in confabulatory delusional states 161
    delusional 98, 111, 125
    flight from, paranoid reactions as 127
    function, Janet's (P.) concept of 192
    Minkowski's (E.), concept of vital
        contact with 188–93
    schizophrenic loss of contact with
        191–3
    see also autism; withdrawal from the
        external world
reasoning, disorders of 170
    delusional development and 7
    in Lacan's (J.) self-punitive paranoia
        223
    in misinterpretative delusional states 7,
        161, 171, 220
reference/self-reference
    déjà vu experiences of 109–10
    delusions of 105–6, 112, 121
    sensitive delusions of 112, 123–4, 137
    see also significance, delusional
        perception of
reflexes in schizophrenia 20, 68
regression to earlier stages of
    development 131–2
Reiss, E., primitive thinking 131
remission
    of schizophrenia 61–2; of individual
        symptoms 69–70; mechanism of
        70–1
    of self-punitive paranoia 224
residual symptoms
    of schizophrenia 16, 21, 70
    of simple schizophrenia 32
    see also dementia, schizophrenic
rigidity
    mental 83, 129
    of perception 93–4
role theory, sociological 139

Scheid, W., on misidentification 100, 109
Scherner, X., dream interpretation 44
Schilder, P., primitive modes of thinking
    99, 131
schizoid personality 2–3
schizomania 200
schizophrenia 59, 150, 190
    Binswanger's existential analysis of
        83–8
    consciousness in, see consciousness,
        disturbances of
    dementia of, see dementia,
        schizophrenic
    dissociation of, see association,
        disturbance of; dissociation between
        and within mental functions;

intrapsychic ataxia; splitting of
    psychic functions
'end of the world experience' 85, 106,
    108–9, 114
familial and sporadic forms 6
French concept of 6
hebephrenic, see hebephrenia
incurability of 61–2
introduction of the term 4, 59
latent 61
Minkowski's theories on the essential
    disorder underlying 188–212
organic nature of: changing views of
    1–2, 5, 130; Kleist's views on 5, 75–8,
    130–1; Kraepelin's views of 23;
    Weygandt's, (W.), theory of 48–50
outcome, assessment of 72–3
perplexity in 79–80
prognosis 59–74; in acute stages 64–5,
    69; in chronic stages 65; concept of
    59–60; distinction between primary
    and secondary symptoms 65–9;
    general and specific 60–1; problems
    in estimation of 71–3
psychoanalytical theories of 4, 45–8, 50
remission, see remission of
    schizophrenia
residual symptoms 16, 21, 70
simple, see simple schizophrenia
spatial thought in 201–12
time-course of 62–3
    see also catatonia; delusions; dementia
        praecox; discordant insanity;
        paranoia
Schmidt, Gerhardt, on delusions 4, 98,
    104–34
Schneider, Carl, on delusions 112–13,
    114, 116
Schneider, Kurt 136
    delusional perception 98, 101, 107–8
    delusions of reference 123, 127
    existential change and 116
    secondary delusions 108, 117
Schulte, H., disordered sense of belong
    ing 124–5
secrecy in misinterpretative delusional
    states 174
sejunction 35–6, 39–40, 41, 55
self, or self-ness, morbid disturbance of
    112
self-accusation, ideas of 173, 181
self-awareness
    depersonalization and 53, 197
    in general paralysis of the insane 197
    see also awareness; depersonalization
self-punitive paranoia (the case of Aimée)
    213–26
self-punitive personality trait 224–6

self-reference, *see* reference/self-reference

senile dementia, differentiation from simple schizophrenia 33

sensitive delusions of reference 122, 123–4, 137

sensitive personality, delusional development in 122, 123–4, 137, 225

Sérieux, Paul, misinterpretative delusional states 7, 167, 168–81, 219

sexual deviation due to delusional states 130

sexual excitement, states of 18

sexuality
delusional development and 130
dreams and 44

significance
compulsive disorders of abnormal ('symbolic awareness') 100–2, 103
delusional perception of 105, 106, 113–14, 120; Matussek on 98–9, 101, 103
see also connections, increased ability to form; reference/self-reference

simple schizophrenia (dementia simplex) 2, 3, 25–34
aetiology 29–30, 34
case histories 25–7
clinical features 27–9
course of illness 30–1, 34
diagnosis and differential diagnosis 32–3

simulation of mental illness, diagnosis of 37–8, 41

skin responses in dementia praecox 20

sleep disturbances in schizophrenia 20, 68

social adequacy, rating of 72

social psychiatry 138, 139, 142

sociology applied to psychiatry 138, 139

somatic introspection 178

spatial disorientation 196–7

spatial thought in schizophrenia 201–12

Specht, G., on suspiciousness 129

speech disorders of schizophrenia 16, 17, 41, 78
arrested development and 49
manifested in organic disorders 75–6, 78
role of thought disorder in 76
see also language

split personality 3, 55–8

splittinig of psychic functions 55, 59, 83, 86
see also association, disturbance of; dissociation between and within mental functions; intraspychic ataxia; discordant insanity

stereotyped symptoms 67, 70, 155

Stoecker, W., 129

Storch, A., on schizophrenic thinking 98, 99, 100, 115, 131–2

Störring, Gustav, views on perplexity 4, 5, 79–82

Stransky, Erwin 3–4, 36, 37–41
intrapsychic ataxia of 4, 37, 39–41, 154, 189–90

Straus, A., 137–8

structuralism 139

stupor 68, 69, 83, 157
assessment in 65
remission of 69

sudden delusional ideas 105, 107–8
mood and 117
types of 109, 110

suspiciousness, as an affect 129

symbolic awareness (or symbolic experience) 100–2, 103

symbolic context 98–9

symptomatic psychoses
delusional perception in 107
perplexity associated with 81–2

Szasz, T., 139

temporal lobe defects, speech disorders in 75–6

temporal lobe epilepsy, psychoses associated with 5

tetany preceding dementia praecox 20

thought
co-ordination, disturbance in 77
disconnectedness 29
disorder 68; alogical 77–8; delusions as a product of 112–13, 114, 116; in mild dementia praecox 14, 16; Minkowski's, (E.), theories on schizophrenic 5, 188–212; in organic disorders 5, 76–8; paralogical 76–7, 78; as a product of delusional mood states 114–15; role in speech disorders 76; in simple schizophrenia 29
insertion, delusions derived from 118
passive, involuntary 52
primitive modes of 99–100, 131–2
see also reasoning, disorders of

thymo-psyche, Stransky's 4, 39, 40

thyroid dysfunction associated with self-punitive paranoia 219, 220

time, loss of sense of 86, 198–9

toxic confusional states, clouding of consciousness in 53

toxic states, delusions of self-reference in 106

tremor of the hands in simple schizophrenia 34

tuberculous meningitis, differentiation from hebephrenia 156

understandability, criterion of 117
understandable explanations of delusions
    120–8
    external conflicts 126–8
    inner conflicts and emotions 124–6
    personality and 120–4
understanding psychology 90, 136, 137
Urstein, M., intrapsychic dysharmony
    154, 190

vagrancy
    in confabulatory delusional states 167
    in mild dementia praecox 16
    in simple schizophrenia 27, 29
vasomotor system, disturbances of 68
verbal insanity, discordant 147, 150–2,
    157
Verblödung, meaning of the term 200
Verstiegenheit, meaning of 86
violent behaviour 20, 28
vital contact with reality, Minkowski's,
    (E.), concept of 188–93
von Baeyer, W. 116, 132, 138
von Domarus, E. 111
von Gebsattel, V. E. 101, 137–8

Wagner, a headmaster with paranoia
    (Gaupp) 120–2
weight, body, changes in 21, 68
Werner, H. 99–100
Wernicke, Carl, 41, 70, 118
    concept of sejunction 36, 39–40, 55

Wesenseigenschaft, meaning of 95
Westerterp, M., 110–11
Wetzel, A., 106, 136
    'end of the world experience' 108–9
    on litiginous paranoia 127
Weygandt, Wilhelm, 33, 42–50
    apperceptive dementia 49, 189
    criticisms of psychoanalytical theories
        4, 42–8, 50
    organic nature of schizophrenia 4,
        48–50
Wieck, H., psychopathometry 140
will, lack of 189, 221
wish fulfilment, paranoid reactions and
    127
'wish reversal' in paranoia 125–6
wishful paranoiac personality type,
    delusional development in 122, 123
withdrawal from the external world
    in normal people 202
    in schizophrenia 69, 70, 81
    see also autism; reality
word amnesias 75
writing in mild dementia praecox 16
Wyrsch, J., 118

'youthful insanity' 22

Ziehen, T., 119
Zucker, K., experience of significance
    113–14
Zutt, J., 111–12, 138